Consultation Skills
for the new MRCGP

Consultation Skills
for the new **MRCGP**

Practice cases for CSA and COT

P. Naidoo
MBChB, MRCGP, DRCOG, DFFP, Dip Occ Med, MSc
GP in Oxfordshire

and

C. Monkley
MBBS, DRCOG, MSc (Sports Medicine),
MRCGP, FFSEM (UK)
GP in the Defence Medical Services

Scion

First published 2009, reprinted 2009, 2010

A CIP catalogue record for this book is available from the British Library.

ISBN 978 1 904842 60 6

Scion Publishing Limited
The Old Hayloft, Vantage Business Park,
Bloxham Road, Banbury, Oxfordshire OX16 9UX
www.scionpublishing.com

Important Note from the Publisher
The information contained within this book was obtained by Scion Publishing Limited from sources believed by us to be reliable. However, while every effort has been made to ensure its accuracy, no responsibility for loss or injury whatsoever occasioned to any person acting or refraining from action as a result of information contained herein can be accepted by the authors or publishers.

The reader should remember that medicine is a constantly evolving science and while the authors and publishers have ensured that all dosages, applications and practices are based on current indications, there may be specific practices which differ between communities. You should always follow the guidelines laid down by the manufacturers of specific products and the relevant authorities in the country in which you are practising.

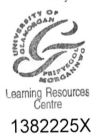

Typeset by Phoenix Photosetting, Chatham, Kent, UK
Printed by Cromwell Press Group, Trowbridge

Contents

Preface

This book is written as a companion guide to *Cases and Concepts for the new MRCGP* (2008). The aim is to help readers pull together the knowledge and communication skills required for success in the consultation components of the new MRCGP exam, namely Clinical Skills Assessment (CSA) and Clinical Observation Tool (COT). The book does this in three ways:

- by demonstrating some of the required consultation skills on the accompanying DVD
- by identifying and teaching these skills in the case write-ups
- by giving candidates 'mock cases' on which to practise, either alone or in small groups

The book and DVD are meant to be interactive. The DVD features 13 GP consultations and readers are asked if the doctor on the DVD:

- asked the right questions, at the right time, in the right way
- performed the right examination correctly
- communicated in a precise, understandable and sensitive manner

In the DVD cases that are marked according to a CSA marking schedule, readers are referred to various sources of information so that they have adequate knowledge to make judgements. In all the cases, additional medical information is provided to clarify the management decisions and justify the weighting of the accompanying marking schedule. If readers feel that the doctor's performance in a particular area is inadequate, they are invited to suggest how they would improve performance. Group work can be quite useful in this regard.

Once candidates learn from the DVD, they are presented with 20 complete cases designed to aid them in CSA preparation and COT discussions. Each of the 20 cases features detailed analysis to demonstrate to candidates an ordered, step-wise approach to data gathering, clinical management and interpersonal skills.

Hence we feel that this book would be useful to Specialist Trainees (ST) in general practice right from the start of their training.

- ST1s will find DVD cases 1–7 most useful.
- ST2s, reading the analysis and discussion in the long cases, will be prepared for COT discussions.
- ST3s preparing for the CSA are directed to DVD cases 8–13 and the final section of the book, Mock Cases, which provides examples of typical CSA questions and focuses on cases not previously covered in *Cases and Concepts for the new MRCGP*. There is greater coverage of paediatric and telephone consultations, dealing with lists, breaking bad news, and home visits.

Good luck with your studying!

Dr P Naidoo and Dr C Monkley
August, 2008

Acknowledgments

Thank you to the patients and staff at my surgery. I enjoy your company and the challenges you present.

Dr Dougie Wyper: now that we've made it to Fairford, Farnborough and Henley, I look forward to new social heights.

Dr Jonathan Ray: thank you for your kind words, hard cash and belief in me.

Finally, to my husband Anton – no, you cannot have Sky Sports!

Dedication

This book is dedicated to my mother who has enjoyed teaching for more than 40 years, a hard act to follow.

Analysing consultation skills: the DVD

The aim of the DVD (attached to the inside back cover) is to model for candidates the communication skills required for effective consultation in the COT and CSA. There are thirteen cases in total. Video cases one to seven are analysed using the COT template. Video cases eight to thirteen are accompanied by a CSA marking grid to give the viewer a chance to assess the doctor's performance.

Each of the 13 video cases comprises the following sections.
- *'Brief to the doctor'*, with a summary of the patient's relevant details, including any recent test results. The 'locum' doctor, like the CSA candidate, is provided with the patient's basic background at the start of clinic.
- *'Tasks for the doctor'*: in video cases one to seven, the doctor is tasked to observe the useful consultation skills this case illustrates and to comment on whether any important aspects of the consultation are omitted. In video cases eight to thirteen, the candidate is informed about the examiner's thought processes, which explains the weighting of the accompanying marking grid.
- *'Approach to be taken'*: a review of the doctor's approach is provided in video cases one to seven, with an explanation of consultation behaviours demonstrated and missed. In video cases eight to thirteen, a CSA marking grid is provided to enable candidates to mark the DVD cases themselves.
- *'Debrief'*: each debrief highlights the communication techniques that can be learnt from the case.
- Each case ends with suggestions for further reading.

Video cases 1–7
- Read through the case's entire write-up before watching the DVD.
- Look at the 'tasks for the doctor when watching the case' so that you are clear about which specific techniques you are cued to observe.
- Watch the case. You may wish to use a COT *pro forma* to help you to 'mark' the doctor's performance. Please remember, marks are given for the doctor's questioning, examination technique and explanation, and not for the patient's contribution.
- Debrief, either alone, or in a group, consolidating the skills learnt from the case.

Video cases 8–13
- Read through the 'patient summary' and 'tasks for the doctor.'
- Refer to the background information provided – this informs the marking grid.
- While watching the DVD, consult the marking grid and tick when positive or negative indicators are demonstrated.
- Make a global judgement by asking if this doctor, based on this consultation, is fit for independent practice.
- Debrief, preferably in a small group.

COT *pro forma*[1]

A. Data gathering, examination and clinical assessment skills

1. **Define the clinical problem:**
    - What questions do you ask to clarify why the patient has presented today?
    - How would you explore the patient's ideas, concerns, expectations and health beliefs?

2. **Perform an appropriate physical or mental examination**
    - What is the appropriate targeted physical or mental state examination?
    - Can you perform the examination slickly and sensitively using appropriate medical equipment?

B. Clinical management skills

3. **Make an appropriate working diagnosis**
    - On the basis of probability, what is your working diagnosis?

4. **Explain the problem to the patient using appropriate language**
    - How would you explain the diagnosis to the patient?
    - Is your explanation jargon-free, well organised and logical?
    - Does it address the patient's concerns and expectations?

5. **Provide holistic care and use resources effectively**
    - Was your management plan informed by national or local guidelines?
    - Have you referred appropriately?

6. **Prescribe appropriately**
    - Have you considered drug interactions or discussed side effects?
    - Did you check the patient's understanding of the medication?

7. **Specify the conditions and interval for follow-up**
    - Have you safety netted appropriately?

---

1   Adapted from a COT *pro forma* developed by Dr David Chadwick, Springfield Surgery, Oxfordshire.

C. Interpersonal skills: know and treat this patient

8. Achieve rapport
- Have you demonstrated active listening, sensitivity, and empathy?
- Have you used the patient's ideas and beliefs in explanations?
- Have you addressed the patient's specific concerns and expectations?

9. Give the patient the opportunity to be involved in significant management decisions
- Have you involved the patient in decisions?
- Have you negotiated, offered various treatment options or encouraged autonomy and opinions?

Video 1 – Knee pain

Brief to the doctor

Miss AS is a 22 year old woman who presents with knee pain.

Patient summary

Name	AS
Date of birth (Age)	22
Past medical history	Contraception
Repeat medication	Microgynon as directed

Tasks for the doctor when watching the case

The tasks are to:
- take note of the verbal and non-verbal communication the doctor employed to put the patient at ease
- notice how the doctor used a mixture of open and closed questions to take a systematic and detailed history
- comment on the fluency of the doctor's examination
- assess whether the examination findings proved or disproved the doctor's suspicions
- assess whether the patient understood the explanation? How could the doctor have simplified the explanation or checked the patient's understanding?

Review of the doctor's approach

A. Data gathering, examination and clinical assessment skills

1. *Define the clinical problem: clarify why the patient has presented today*
   The doctor:
   - leaned forward, smiled, made good eye contact and nodded appropriately, thereby establishing good rapport
   - asked open questions to explore the problem, such as *"how can I help?"* and *"describe the pain?"*
   - asks closed questions to clarify details about the knee pain: *"do you get pain at other times? Is there giving way? Locking? Is there pain on walking up or down the stairs? Have you injured the knee? Are there problems with other joints?"*

- explored the patient's health understanding by asking *"have you thought about what this might be?"*
- explored the patient's concerns: *"is there anything you are worried about?"*

The doctor could have:
- gained more information on how the knee pain was affecting her job or her activities at home. He could have enquired whether her inability to train affected her interactions with work colleagues.

2. *Performs an appropriate physical or mental examination*
   - The knee was examined; hence the examination was appropriate and directed.

The doctor could have:
- asked the patient if she preferred to have a chaperone present
- made the examination more fluent and systematic, following the 'look, feel and move' approach to joint examination

B. Clinical management skills

3. *Make an appropriate working diagnosis*
   - The doctor made a working diagnosis of 'problem with the tendon at the knee cap.'
   - The case was written to be patello-femoral pain, secondary to excessive foot pronation.

4. *Explain the problem to the patient using appropriate language*
   The doctor:
   - attempted to explain the diagnosis to the patient using phrases such as *"the ligaments are intact"* and *"there is no fluid in the knee"*
   - prescribed ibuprofen and paracetamol appropriately and the doctor specifically asked if the patient knew what the maximum dosages were, thus demonstrating an attempt to enhance concordance

   However, the doctor:
   - used words such as 'cartilage', 'tendon', 'inflammation' without clarification and the assessor is not sure if the language used was 'appropriate', particularly as the doctor did not specifically confirm the patient's understanding of the diagnosis
   - did not give the patient the opportunity to be involved in the management plan, although it is entirely appropriate to prescribe pain medication and refer to physiotherapy

5. *Provide holistic care and use resources effectively*
   The doctor:
   - was informed by guidelines (www.emedicine.com/ and search for 'patellofemoral syndrome')

However, the assessor is unsure if:

- holistic care was provided: the issue of training for a marathon was not addressed
- resources were used effectively as the patient's views on taking medication and attending physiotherapy were not sought

6. *Prescribe appropriately*
   The doctor:

   - checked the patient's understanding of the amounts of medication required

7. *Specify the conditions and interval for follow-up*
   The doctor could have:

   - highlighted the importance of proper assessments for suitable footwear
   - specified when he would like to review the patient again, such as *"I expect this condition to improve with physiotherapy but if you make little progress, please see me again"*

C. Interpersonal skills: know and treat this patient

8. *Achieve rapport*
   The doctor:

   - listened attentively to the patient's description of her problem
   - spoke when she stopped – the consultation had a natural cadence
   - empathised with her difficulties in training for the marathon
   - asked if there was anything further the patient required at the end of the consultation

9. *Give the patient the opportunity to be involved in significant management decisions*
   The doctor could have:

   - encouraged autonomy by asking what the patient thought of physiotherapy or non-steroidals

Debrief

- What could you learn from this consultation? How to
  - establish rapport
  - take a systematic and focused history
  - explore the patient's health understanding
  - take steps to enhance concordance
  - be efficient with time
- What questions could you ask to discover the patient's ideas and expectations?
- How would you examine the knee?
- How could you explain the diagnosis of patello-femoral syndrome to the patient?
- How could you involve the patient in the management plan?

Relevant literature

For an excellent website detailing the examination of the knee, with video-clips, see http://medicine.ucsd.edu/clinicalmed/Joints.html

For information on patello-femoral syndrome, see www.emedicine.com/pmr/topic101.htm

Video 2 – Unhappy with last consultation

Brief to the doctor

Mrs SW is a 31 year old woman who saw Dr Brown 2 weeks ago. She is unhappy with her last consultation.

Patient summary

Name	SW
Date of birth (Age)	31
Social and Family History	Married, no children
Past medical history	Sprained ankle 3 years ago
Repeat medication	Marvelon as directed

Consultation note by Dr Brown (2 weeks ago):
'Long list of minor symptoms. Thinks she has diabetes. Urine dipstix negative for glucose. Reassured no diabetes.'

Tasks for the doctor when watching the case

The tasks are to:

- notice how the doctor used open questions to gather a lot of data, followed by summarising to highlight the main problems and indicate to the patient that the doctor had a good grasp of the pertinent issues – this communication style allowed the doctor to structure the consultation
- notice that the open questions were neutral, for example, *"What do you think he did to make you feel like that?"* The non-judgmental questioning style enabled the doctor to obtain information without defending or undermining Dr Brown.
- take note of the doctor's response to an important cue – the patient, early in the consultation, mentioned that symptoms interfered with work; the doctor jotted down the cue, continued with her line of questioning, but a few minutes later asked how the symptoms interfered with work
- comment on how the patient's ideas (on the cause of diabetes), concerns (about a missed early diagnosis) and expectations (of better testing) were elicited

Review of the doctor's approach

A. Data gathering, examination and clinical assessment skills

1. Define the clinical problem: clarify why the patient has presented today
The doctor:
- established good rapport by greeting the patient at the door, smiling, and inviting her to sit
- summarised the history at intervals thereby indicating active listening
- asked open questions to explore the problem, such as *"when you say excessive, what do you mean? Are there any other symptoms? What happens to you when you get irritable?"*
- asked closed questions to assess the likelihood of diabetes: *"are you passing more urine? Are you tired? Have you lost weight?"*
- obtained important information about the patient's family history, which led to a deeper understanding of her concerns
- obtained information about her feelings regarding her work as a dental nurse, which may account for her irritability – dissatisfaction with work is noted as a differential diagnosis but is not offered to the patient as a possibility on this occasion
- explored the patient's health understanding by asking *"what made you suspect diabetes?"*
- explored the patient's concerns: *"What's raising your concerns?"*
- explored the patient's expectations: *"Would you like to talk to Dr Brown? Are you happy for me to have a quiet word with Dr Brown?"*

2. Performs an appropriate physical or mental examination
- The patient was questioned about sleep, tiredness and weight loss, which are also depressive symptoms.

The doctor could have:
- formally assessed BP and weight

B. Clinical management skills

3. Make an appropriate working diagnosis
- The doctor made a working diagnosis of a dissatisfied patient who may have diabetes mellitus.
- The case was written as an angry patient who threatens to complain. Not all her symptoms suggest diabetes and there is some doubt about the likelihood of this diagnosis.

4. Explain the problem to the patient using appropriate language
The doctor could have:
- provided more in the way of explanation of each problem

5. *Provide holistic care and use resources effectively*
The doctor:

- was informed by guidelines: http://cks.library.nhs.uk/diabetes_glycaemic_control/making_a_diagnosis and http://cks.library.nhs.uk/information_for_patients/common_health_questions/question/how_do_i_make_a_complaint_about_my_doctor
- tackled both issues and so provided holistic care; the doctor created a reasonable relationship with the patient to enable on-going care
- made cost-effective use of resources by requesting a fasting blood glucose rather than a GTT

6. *Prescribe appropriately*

- The doctor did not prescribe, which was appropriate in this case.

7. *Specify the conditions and interval for follow-up*
The doctor:

- arranged a fasting blood test

The doctor could have:

- specified a time-scale for the bloods and arranged a follow-up appointment to review the results

C. Interpersonal skills: know and treat this patient

8. *Achieve rapport*
The doctor:

- actively listened and summarised
- regularly checked understanding – in doing so, she refrained from offering superfluous advice on how to formalise a complaint and potential lifestyle changes
- chose not to challenge an angry patient on their first meeting and concentrated instead on establishing a cordial professional relationship
- explored the patient's concerns about early diabetes and addressed her expectations for better testing

9. *Give the patient the opportunity to be involved in significant management decisions*
The doctor:

- offered ways in which the patient could act on her feelings towards Dr Brown

The doctor could have:

- discussed the different diagnostic tests for diabetes and offered the patient a choice; however, this needs to be balanced against risking a longer consultation and justifying the cost of a GGT

Debrief

What could you learn from this consultation? How to
- summarise – to indicate active listening and to structure the consultation
- obtain a psycho-social history
- explore the patient's ideas, concerns and expectations
- be non-judgmental
- deal with two important issues within ten minutes

Summary of learning

Write your answers in the space provided.
1. *What questions would you ask to explore the differential diagnosis?*

2. *What would you say to the patient to involve her in the management plan?*

3. *How could you specify review or follow-up?*

4. *If the patient were unaware of the complaints procedure, how would you explain it to her?*

Relevant literature

Jain A, Ogden J (1999) A qualitative study of general practitioners' experiences of a patient complaint. *BMJ*; **318**: 1596–1599 (www.bmj.com/cgi/content/abstract/318/7198/1596)

http://cks.library.nhs.uk/diabetes_glycaemic_control/making_a_diagnosis

http://cks.library.nhs.uk/information_for_patients/common_health_questions/question/how_do_i_make_a_complaint_about_my_doctor

Video 3 – Pregnant and worried

Brief to the doctor

Mrs GP is a 28 year old woman who has recently registered with your practice. She is pregnant and has seen the midwife for two routine checks.

Patient summary

Name   GP

Date of birth (Age)   28

Social and Family History   Married, 1st pregnancy

Past medical history   Eczema

Repeat medication   Diprobase as directed

Tasks for the doctor when watching the case

The tasks are to:
- notice how the doctor barely spoke at the start of the consultation – this allowed the patient to air her fears and get her concerns off her chest – which in a consultation about social or emotional issues can be therapeutic in itself
- notice how the doctor summarised the patient's presenting problem and highlighted three main issues; the overt structure enabled systematic questioning and explanation
- notice how the doctor interrupted the patient at several points, without annoying the patient. The interruptions occurred at points in the consultation when the patient repeated herself. The interruptions redirected the patient to the main issues. The doctor was able to gather, in the time provided, sufficient data to explore the reasons for the patient's fears and to 'objectively' assess her risk of harm.
- see how the doctor identified the benefits of the patient disclosing her fears to her husband. The patient felt unable to initiate the conversation with her husband, but the doctor suggested a strategy to overcome this barrier, thereby moving the consultation forward.
- notice that, although a good therapeutic relationship was established and follow-up offered, alternative sources of support, such as the midwife, were not suggested
- comment on the doctor's decision to neither prescribe nor refer
- comment on whether sufficient information about the patient's support network or the husband's job stresses was obtained to inform the risk assessment

Review of the doctor's approach

A. Data gathering, examination and clinical assessment skills

1. *Define the clinical problem: clarify why the patient has presented today*
   The doctor:
   - established good rapport by actively listening and by using the patient's words and terminology in questioning and explanations
   - reflected and summarised the history
   - made systematic enquiries along three defined strands
   - asked open questions to explore the problem, such as *"what makes you think he is distant? What do you think is causing that distance? What makes you think he is not interested in the baby?"*
   - asked closed questions to assess the likelihood of harm to the patient: *"did he ask you to have a termination? Did he come with you to the scans? He hasn't got a history of violence, has he?"*
   - obtained information about the husband's occupation; however, the cue about him being in the military was not followed up by questions about the patient's social support (such as whether she is living away from family) or the husband's work pressures
   - obtained important 'red flag' information about her husband's character, whether he was aggressive or had a history of violence, but alcohol or drug use was not queried
   - uncovered the patient's concern about her husband's attitude potentially affecting the baby and explored the reasons for that concern, i.e. the newspaper article about a man who fed his partner 'abortion' pills and killed her baby
   - satisfied the patient's stated expectation (*"I've come for a chat"*). The chat served two purposes: first, it helped the patient to make sense of her feelings, and, secondly, the doctor made offers of help. Hence, the patient was empowered to deal with the problem.

2. *Performs an appropriate physical or mental examination*
   - An examination was not undertaken.

B. Clinical management skills

3. *Make an appropriate working diagnosis*
   - The doctor made a working diagnosis of there being a difference between the expectation and reality of the husband's feelings and behaviours towards the pregnancy, however, this was not pathological.
   - The case was written as about an expectant mum who, after reading a newspaper article about a man who fed his partner 'abortion pills', works herself up into an almost irrational fear for her baby. The doctor needed

to assess her risk of harm. If the risk was assessed incorrectly, the doctor may have made unnecessary referrals or prescribed inappropriately. If the doctor failed to 'listen' to the patient's concerns, she would have felt patronised and become tearful.

4. *Explain the problem to the patient using appropriate language*
   - The doctor spoke about there being a spectrum of reactions to fatherhood. While everyday language was used, the word 'horrible' failed to convey the same meaning as 'pathological'. Perhaps the word 'criminal' would have been more appropriate.

5. *Provide holistic care and use resources effectively*
   The doctor:
   - dealt with a social and emotional issue in a sensitive and constructive manner, hence holistic care was provided. The doctor created a reasonable relationship with the patient to enable on-going care.

   However, the doctor did not:
   - signpost to alternative sources of support, such as the midwife or local volunteer agencies; in the military, the padre also provides pastoral support and counselling

6. *Prescribe appropriately*
   - The doctor did not prescribe, which was appropriate in this case.

7. *Specify the conditions and interval for follow-up*
   - The doctor and patient agreed to meet again if needed.

C. Interpersonal skills: know and treat this patient

8. *Achieve rapport*
   The doctor:
   - actively listened and summarised: *"it seems to me that ..."*
   - checked agreement at several points: *"do you feel happy to have that conversation?"*
   - understood the patient's reaction to the newspaper article; by being supportive, empathetic but detached, the doctor helped the patient to achieve insight and perspective

9. *Give the patient the opportunity to be involved in significant management decisions*
   - The doctor made offers: *"do you feel happy to have that conversation? Do you think you would be able to take this first step more easily now?"*

Debrief

What could you learn from this consultation? How to
- reflect and summarise, using the phrase: *"it seems to me ..."*
- move the consultation forward: after gathering the relevant data, formulate a management plan that empowers the patient
- make offers and check agreement
- deal with challenging social and emotional issues within ten minutes

Summary of learning

Write your answers in the space provided.

1. *What questions would you ask to assess the patient's risk of harm from her husband?*

2. *How would you explain the problem to the patient using words she is likely to understand?*

3. *What would your management plan be? How would you explain the plan to the patient?*

4. *If the patient was socially isolated (living away from family and had not made friends at the military base) and her husband had a history of alcohol binge drinking, would your management change? Justify your decision.*

Relevant literature

For the original article read by the patient, follow *The Guardian* link:
http://lifeandhealth.guardian.co.uk/women/story/0,,2270135,00.html

This was a challenging consultation about a social and emotional issue. If the doctor felt overwhelmed by the patient's presentation, one approach would be to structure the consultation using a consultation model. In this case, the Calgary–Cambridge approach was used. To revise consultation models, see: www.skillscascade.com/models.htm

Video 4 – Repeat script and husband snores

Brief to the doctor

Mrs PB is a 42 year old woman who presents with two problems: first, she requests a repeat prescription of her contraceptive pill, and secondly, she wants to explore what can be done to help her husband's snoring.

Patient summary

Name	PB
Date of birth (Age)	42
Past medical history	Non-focal migraine on combined oral contraception
Repeat medication	Cerazette, one tablet daily x 126

Tasks for the doctor when watching the case

The tasks are to:
- take note of how the doctor explored both agendas within the allocated time
- notice how the doctor gathered sufficient data to prescribe safely
- observe how the doctor communicated the risks and benefits of the Mirena intra-uterine system (IUS) in a way that was meaningful to the patient
- comment on the doctor's non-verbal communication: posture, use of hands, facial expressions
- assess whether the patient felt empowered by the advice she was given on treatments for snoring
- evaluate whether the patient was given the opportunity to be involved in the management plan

Review of the doctor's approach

A. Data gathering, examination and clinical assessment skills

1. *Define the clinical problem: clarify why the patient has presented today*
   The doctor:
   - made good eye contact, nodded appropriately, and encouraged the patient to talk; however, questions such as *"is that what you wanted to talk about today?"* and *"is that alright?"* discouraged a deeper exploration of the main issue, namely marital strain to which snoring was one of many contributing factors.
   - asked open questions to explore the problem, such as *"how are you getting on with [cerazette]?"* and *"how about the migraine side of things?"*
   - asked closed questions to clarify details about the snoring: *"is this placing a strain on your relationship? Have you discussed this with him?"*

   The doctor could have:
   - gained more information about how the snoring affected the patient and her marital relationship by asking neutral questions. When the doctor attempted to explore the patient's irritability and grumpiness, he attributed her feelings to a low mood, and the patient corrected him by saying her feelings were due to her husband's snoring rather than an intrinsic mood disorder. The patient may have felt that the doctor was jumping to the wrong conclusions and consequently may not have felt that the doctor had truly listened to her concerns.
   - explored the patient's health understanding by asking about what had lead her to believe that an operation for her husband's snoring would be the solution to their marriage difficulties. The doctor did not respond to the verbal cue: *"you hear about ops"*
   - identified and addressed the patient's frustrations with not being able to persuade her husband to seek help. It seemed that she was canvassing the doctor for written information about snoring treatments but these expectations were neither acknowledged nor met.

2. *Performs an appropriate physical or mental examination*
   An examination was not essential.

B. Clinical management skills

3. *Make an appropriate working diagnosis*
   - The doctor made a working diagnosis of 'safe to repeat the prescription for the progestogen-only pill (POP), and husband snores, probably due to recent weight gain.'
   - The case was written about the hidden agenda, with the marital difficulties being the real reason for the consultation. The patient, at several points

during the consultation, stressed that she was happy with her Pill. She pulled a face when alternative contraception was discussed, a cue that this was not her primary concern. However, when talking about her husband's snoring, she volunteered information about a *"recent fight"* and described her frustration with her inability to find a solution to the problem of his snoring. She was stuck and wanted help with the snoring problem.

4. *Explain the problem to the patient using appropriate language*
The doctor:
- explored whether the POP was a reasonable and safe contraceptive choice prior to prescribing
- offered long-acting contraception alternatives, in line with NICE guidance
- offered to see the patient's husband and volunteered information on treatments for snoring, namely weight reduction and operations on the palette

However, the doctor:
- used words such as 'palette' and 'oestrogen' without explanation and the assessor is not sure if the language used was 'appropriate' to the patient's understanding. The patient, having already asked if it was OK to broach the subject of her husband's snoring (*"do we have time to talk about another issue?"*), may not have volunteered her lack of understanding.
- in prescribing the POP, did not demonstrate an attempt to enhance concordance

5. *Provide holistic care and use resources effectively*
The doctor:
- addressed both issues (contraception and snoring)
- was informed by guidelines: www.nice.org.uk/guidance/index.jsp?action=byID&o=10974

However, the assessor is unsure if:
- holistic care was provided: the issue of snoring was superficially explored, and so it was difficult to move the problem forward. Had the doctor uncovered the patient's true concerns and expectations, the doctor could have designed a more inclusive and holistic management plan.
- the patient left the consultation armed with new information that could persuade her husband to see his GP. Hence marks cannot be awarded for 'empowering the patient.'

6. *Prescribe appropriately*
The doctor could have:
- checked the patient's understanding of the amounts of medication required and asked if she had a family planning booklet for written advice on 'missed pills' and commonly occurring pill interactions

7. *Specify the conditions and interval for follow-up*
The doctor could have:

- signposted the patient to information on treatments for snoring or given a leaflet detailing the medical help available
- specified when he would like to review the patient again, such as by saying *"I have given you a prescription for a six month supply of the Pill. Please see me or the practice nurse for a review in six months"*.

C. Interpersonal skills: know and treat this patient

8. *Achieve rapport*
The doctor:

- listened attentively to the patient's description of her two presenting problems
- reflected appropriately: *"is this putting a strain on your relationship?"*
- asked if there was anything further the patient required at the end of the consultation: *"is that alright?"*

9. *Give the patient the opportunity to be involved in significant management decisions*
The doctor could have:

- encouraged the patient's involvement in the management plan: *"I have suggested your husband come and see us for weight loss advice and for further information on operations for snoring. What do you think about this plan?"*

Debrief

- What could you learn from this consultation? How to
  - take a systematic and focused history for safe POP prescribing
  - address two issues in 10 minutes
  - be efficient with time (by avoiding unnecessary examinations)
- What questions could you ask to discover the patient's concerns and expectations?
- How would you explore the issue of the husband's snoring?
- How could you briefly outline long-acting contraceptive alternatives to the patient?
- How could you involve the patient in the management plan?

Relevant literature

For an excellent overview of various contraceptive choices, see www.youtube.com – search for 'Contraception Owens' for a video-clip by Annette Owens.

For information on long-acting contraception, see www.nice.org.uk/guidance/index.jsp?action=byID&o=10974.

For an overview of initial treatments for snoring see www.youtube.com – search for 'snoring + advice' for a video-clip from a Good Morning Texas broadcast.

19

Video 5 – Infertility

Brief to the doctor

Mrs CD is a 28 year old woman who presents with difficulty in conceiving.

Patient summary

Name	CD
Date of birth (Age)	28
Past medical history	Nil of significance
Repeat medication	None for the last year

Tasks for the doctor when watching the case

The tasks are to:

- take note of the 'wait time', that is the length of the pause, or the time taken for the doctor to make the shift from listening to the patient to questioning her (for a detailed explanation of 'wait time', see 'attentive listening' at www.commscascade. medschl.cam.ac.uk/pages/whatteach.html)
- comment on how the doctor signalled to the patient to continue telling her story. Look at the use of head nods, facial expression and neutral facilitative comments such as *"uh-huh"*, *"right"* and *"I see"*.
- assess the doctor's tone, rate and volume of speech and comment on its impact on the consultation
- comment on the doctor's ability to phrase and deliver information about investigation for infertility in a way the patient was able to understand
- assess whether the information given was needed or wanted
- assess whether the doctor checked to see how the patient was reacting to what she said?

Review of the doctor's approach

A. Data gathering, examination and clinical assessment skills

1. *Define the clinical problem: clarify why the patient has presented today*
   The doctor:
   - invited the patient into the room, smiled warmly, sat facing the patient, nodded appropriately, and paused after the patient spoke thereby signalling a willingness to listen and encouraging the patient to tell her story
   - asked reflective questions, using the patient's words and phrasing, such as *"some time?"* and *"when you thought of a referral?"*
   - after establishing the reason for the patient's attendance, progressed to the data gathering section of the consultation using sign-posting and transitional statements, such as *"I don't know you. I'm going to ask you quite a few questions to see how I can best help you."* The transfer from an open to closed style of questioning was made clear to the patient – signposted. As this was done explicitly, the patient was not disturbed by the change in questioning style.
   - asked closed questions to clarify details about the gynaecological history: *"do you have gynae problems? Pelvic infection? Pelvic or abdominal surgery?"*
   - explored the patient's expectations by asking *"when you came in, what were you hoping to get from this consultation? When you thought of a referral, were there any tests you had in mind?"*
   - explored the patient's concerns: *"how do you feel about [the guidelines for referral in the UK being different to the Australian guidance]?"*

   The doctor could have:
   - gained more social and psychological information such as whether the patient came from a large family or whether there was any expectation from her husband or family for her to become pregnant quickly

2. *Performs an appropriate physical or mental examination*
   - Prior to requesting blood tests, the doctor checked for pallor. The examination was targeted, that is, if pallor was noted, it would be appropriate to request a FBC

   The doctor could have:
   - taken her BP

21

B. Clinical management skills

3. *Make an appropriate working diagnosis*
   - The doctor made a working diagnosis of 'difficulty conceiving; no indication for early fertility clinic referral in a woman under 35 years'.
   - The case was written to be difficulty conceiving, in a well-informed health care worker (pharmacist) who has read widely around the topic on the internet.

4. *Explain the problem to the patient using appropriate language*
   The doctor:
   - explained the UK fertility referral guidelines to the patient using reassuring statements and humour
   - provided the correct amount and type of information
   - involved the patient – shared thinking, explained rationale, explained why some blood tests (and not others) were requested

5. *Provide holistic care and use resources effectively*
   The doctor:
   - was informed by guidelines (http://cks.library.nhs.uk/infertility#-296878)
   - provided holistic care by addressing issues such as regular sexual intercourse, folic acid intake, cervical smears, and lifestyle
   - used resources effectively, requesting appropriate and targeted blood tests

   However, chlamydia screening was not discussed.

6. *Prescribe appropriately*
   The doctor:
   - appropriately chose not to prescribe

7. *Specify the conditions and interval for follow-up*
   The doctor:
   - advised the patient to make an appointment for non-fasting blood tests

   The doctor could have:
   - arranged for chlamydia screening for both partners
   - offered to see the husband for a general health check and consultation
   - arranged for semen analysis

C. Interpersonal skills: know and treat this patient

8. *Achieve rapport*
   The doctor:
   - used 'wait time' effectively – her pauses gave the patient time to think, to contribute more, and to speak for longer; the doctor needed to ask fewer questions to extract the important information
   - spoke slowly, looked interested and made good eye contact signalling her interest in the patient's problem and her willingness to help

9. *Give the patient the opportunity to be involved in significant management decisions*
The doctor:
- encouraged autonomy by asking the patient if blood tests were something she'd be interested in; she involved the patient in the management plan

Debrief

- What could you learn from this consultation? How to:
  - take an accurate, systematic and focused clinical history
  - weave in the patient's framework
  - build the relationship with the patient
  - explain, give information and plan without repetition
  - devise a joint management plan that is acceptable to the patient
- How would you negotiate the decision not to refer with the patient?
- How would you encourage the patient to persuade her husband to attend?

Relevant literature

For an excellent website on consultation skills, see www.commscascade.medschl.cam.ac.uk/

For information on infertility, see www.emedicine.com/med/topic3535.htm

Video 6 – Domestic violence

Brief to the doctor

Miss SB is a 23 year old woman who has recently moved to the local area after her partner was posted on to the neighbouring military base. Her notes have not arrived as yet. This is her first consultation and she presents with domestic violence.

Patient summary

The medical record has not arrived into your practice as yet.

Tasks for the doctor when watching the case

The tasks are to:

- evaluate how the doctor enabled and encouraged the doctor–patient partnership
- notice how the doctor promoted openness and trust to facilitate mutual decision-making
- comment on the doctor's decision not to exchange information with outside agencies
- assess whether the doctor responded flexibly to the patient's expectations and needs
- evaluate whether the doctor created a therapeutic relationship in which the patient could be supported over a period of time

Review of the doctor's approach

A. Data gathering, examination and clinical assessment skills

1. *Define the clinical problem: clarify why the patient has presented today*
   The doctor:
   - demonstrated acceptance, that is, she accepted non-judgmentally what the patient said. By accepting the patients' ideas and emotions without initially interrogating or dissuading her, she acknowledged the patient's position and feelings.
   - demonstrated empathy; this was achieved in several ways: she matched her tone of voice to the patient's, she did less of the talking, and she refrained from dispensing advice
   - picked up on the patient's confusion over who was to blame for the violence, tentatively explored the issue, and then reassured with sensitivity

- asked open questions to explore the problem, such as *"what is the situation at the moment?"* and *"what violence has there been?"*
- asked closed questions to clarify details about the domestic violence: *"was that a significant injury? Do you have any children? Are you financially dependent on him? Have you spoken to him?"*
- explored the patient's ideas: *"Are you feeling as if it's your fault?"*
- explored the patient's concerns by asking *"what will happen if you stay?"*
- explored the patient's expectations: *"would you like me to refer you to somebody? What about a drop-in centre?"*

The doctor could have:
- gained more information on the patient's support network, such as the physical distance away from family and friends, and whether her partner also frightened them – this is important should she require refuge from her current living situation
- asked about the partner's alcohol or drug use, and whether or not he had a criminal record

2. *Performs an appropriate physical or mental examination*
- A formal examination was not required.

B. Clinical management skills

3. *Make an appropriate working diagnosis*
- The doctor made a working diagnosis of 'domestic violence, mainly emotional and psychological but also physical'
- The case was written to be domestic violence in a young socially isolated woman who is beginning to believe that she is somehow to blame and who is uncertain about leaving because of economic and emotional repercussions.

4. *Explain the problem to the patient using appropriate language*
The doctor:
- explained that abused women are often made to feel that they are somehow to blame
- gave an explanation that was concise and understandable
- did not give advice or reassure prematurely

5. *Provide holistic care and use resources effectively*
The doctor:
- was informed by guidelines (RCGP, Domestic violence: the general practitioner's role: www.rcgp.org.uk/Default.aspx?page=2259)
- encouraged the patient to contribute her preferences for treatment by asking: *"what would you like to do about this?"*
- involved the patient by making suggestions (about referrals, involving outside agencies or looking on the internet) rather than directing the

patient to what the doctor thought was best. By offering choices, a mutually acceptable plan was negotiated. Had the initial plan (of referral) not been checked with the patient, the barriers to successful treatment (boyfriend checking mail and texts) would not have been addressed.

- safety netted by offering her realistic choices for follow-up while accepting that the decisions regarding treatment were hers alone

However, the assessor is unsure if:

- the patient was offered help in contacting any of the suggested agencies, such as the local women's aid refuge, local authority social services department, or the Department of Social Security
- the patient was advised on how to plan for an emergency, of a financial or personal safety nature

6. *Prescribe appropriately*
- The doctor, appropriately, did not prescribe.

7. *Specify the conditions and interval for follow-up*
The doctor:
- signposted the patient to appropriate information
- suggested to the patient that she would like to *"meet up"* again – it was more appropriate to make an offer than to contract follow up

C. Interpersonal skills: know and treat this patient

8. *Achieve rapport*
The doctor:
- was not judgmental
- communicated her understanding and appreciation of the patient's predicament (*"if he doesn't know what will make him happy, how could you know?"*)
- provided support: expressed concern, understanding and willingness to help (*"This sounds like an awful situation. You don't sound very hopeful"*)
- dealt sensitively with a disturbing topic

9. *Give the patient the opportunity to be involved in significant management decisions*
The doctor:
- shared thinking with the patient to encourage her involvement (*"it seems to me that you are in the process of exploring your options"*)
- offered options – her efforts were directed towards enabling the patient to make the decisions best suited to her personal circumstances

Debrief

- What could you learn from this consultation? How to:
  - discuss a difficult topic with sensitivity
  - support the patient
  - tactfully offer an opinion of what is going on
  - be efficient with time
- What questions could you ask to explore what support she has available from family and friends?
- If she had a bruise on her hand, would you examine her? To what extent?
- How could you explain the rationale and purpose of your examination to her?
- If she disclosed that she was concerned about the safety of her child, how would your management plan change? What would you say to her?

Relevant literature

Dr Iona Heath (RCGP) *Domestic violence: the general practitioner's role*, available on-line: www.rcgp.org.uk/Default.aspx?page=2259

For information on acceptance and empathy, see:
www.gp-training.net/training/communication_skills/calgary/rapport.htm

Video 7 – Chest pain

Brief to the doctor

Ms TR is a 60 year old woman who presents with chest pain. She has registered as a temporary patient. She lives in Austria and is visiting her grandchildren in the UK. She wants to know if she is fit to fly to Austria tomorrow.

Patient summary

Name	TR
Date of birth (Age)	60
Past medical history	None recorded
Repeat medication	None recorded

Tasks for the doctor when watching the case

The tasks are to:
- take note of how the doctor assessed the patient's ideas, concerns and expectations within the opening minutes of the consultation
- notice how the doctor signposted the patient to the history taking, warning her that she was about to ask several questions about the condition and risk factors for heart disease
- comment on the choice of the doctor's examination – she took the pulse, BP, auscultated the heart and examined the neck veins. Would you have done a more or less detailed examination? What would you examine and why?
- did the patient appear to understand the explanation? If yes, what made the explanation easy to understand? If no, what would you do to improve the explanation? What words would you use?
- Notice how the doctor safety-netted (GTN prescription and letter to Austrian GP). Do you think this is adequate? Should the doctor have advised the patient to warn the airline or ask for oxygen?
- Would you have requested a baseline ECG or a pin-prick haemoglobin? Justify your answer.

Review of the doctor's approach

A. Data gathering, examination and clinical assessment skills

1. *Define the clinical problem: clarify why the patient has presented today*
   The doctor:
   - hardly spoke during the 'Golden Minute' – she simply facilitated disclosure in the 1st minute by nodding her head and saying *"right"*
   - responded to the patient's cue with *"you look a bit worried"*
   - elicited the patient's concerns: *"What are you hoping this won't be?"*
   - signposted the patient to the raft of open and closed questions she was about to ask about the chest pain and risk factors for heart disease
   - used explorative questions such as *"what happens at the top of the hill?"* and *"what made you give up [smoking]?"*
   - used closed questions to clarify details: *"How many times did you get pain? Do you suffer from hypertension?"*
   - prefaced the examination by saying *"there's still a bit we don't know. Let's examine you first..."*

   The doctor could have:
   - gained more psycho-social information about how the patient was *"coping with all this? Is it having an effect on the visit?"*
   - asked whether the patient was concerned about flying with the pain. Did the patient want to know if she should inform the airline or change her travel arrangements?

2. *Performs an appropriate physical or mental examination*
   - The pulse, BP, chest and neck veins were examined; hence the examination was appropriate and directed.
   - The doctor said to the patient *"you have a fantastic BP. Is that due to exercise?"*

   According to Sign Guidance (2001):
   - weight, height, body mass index, and waist circumference should be measured
   - evidence of hyperlipidaemia (e.g. xanthelasma, tendon xanthomata), vascular disease (e.g. absent foot pulses, bruits) anaemia or hyperthyroidism should be sought

   For fitness to fly with stable angina, the patient should not have a Hb <7.5 g/dl.

   What examinations would you do? Comment on the fluency of your technique.

B. Clinical management skills

3. *Make an appropriate working diagnosis*
   - Prior to launching into an explanation, the doctor asked *"what do you know about angina?"*.
   - The doctor explained angina simply using language – pictures or leaflets were not used.
   - The case was written to be the initial presentation of stable angina in a temporary resident who is needs an urgent assessment of fitness to fly. The doctor has to decide which examination and investigations need to be undertaken urgently to inform the risk assessment for fitness to fly. Decisions regarding travel and medication need to be made in the face of uncertainty.

4. *Explain the problem to the patient using appropriate language*
   The doctor:
   - attempted to explain the diagnosis to the patient using phrases such as *"furring of the blood vessels"* and *"increased work of the heart"*
   - prescribed GTN spray appropriately (the British Airways website advises that patients with angina may fly and asks them to remember to carry their medication on their person).

5. *Provide holistic care and use resources effectively*
   The doctor:
   - was informed by guidelines (www.sign.ac.uk/pdf/sign96.pdf)
   - provided holistic care: the issue of fitness to fly was addressed and the patient was asked *"how do you feel about flying tomorrow?"*
   - used resources effectively: the doctor offered to post a letter to the patient or her GP, outlining the discussion today and leaving future investigations (blood tests and stress ECG) up to the clinician with overall responsibility for the patient's care

   However, the assessor is unsure:
   - if sufficient data were gathered (emotional precipitants for chest pain, anaemia and exclusion of baseline ECG changes) to inform a through risk assessment. The case was written such that if the doctor asked for a baseline ECG, the patient would have handed over a copy of the ECG saying the triage nurse *"thought you may want this"*.

6. *Prescribe appropriately*
   The doctor:
   - prescribed GTN spray as an interim measure should anything happen on the flight
   - asked *"do you know about GTN sprays"*

7. *Specify the conditions and interval for follow-up*
The doctor:
- advised the patient to see her GP to organise further investigation

However, the assessor is unsure that:
- the patient understood the time-scale in which this should be done

C. Interpersonal skills: know and treat this patient

8. *Achieve rapport*
The doctor:
- listened attentively to the patient's description of her problem
- recognised the patient's concern that she may have a heart problem
- asked if she had answered her queries about medication, flying and ability to organise further tests through her GP in Austria

9. *Give the patient the opportunity to be involved in significant management decisions*
The doctor:
- encouraged autonomy by asking whether the patient felt more comfortable taking or not taking the GTN spray on to the flight. Had the patient said she was uncomfortable, then the reasons for this could have been explored and addressed.

Debrief

- What could you learn from this consultation? How to:
  - facilitate information gathering in the 'Golden Minute'
  - signpost prior to taking a systematic and focused history
  - decide which examinations to perform to inform your risk assessment
  - explain conditions in simple language, avoiding jargon
  - be efficient with resources
- How would you assess the patient's fitness to fly?
- How would you examine the cardiovascular system?
- How would you involve the patient in the management plan?

Relevant literature

For an excellent website detailing the examination of the heart, with links to heart sounds, see: http://meded.ucsd.edu/clinicalmed/heart.htm

For information on fitness to fly with medical conditions, see www.britishairways.com/travel/healthmedcond/public/en_gb#medical and http://whqlibdoc.who.int/publications/2005/9241580364_chap2.pdf

For a useful consultation guide, see www.pennine-gp-training.co.uk/Useful-phrases-for-achieving-COT-competencies.doc

Video 8 – Pregnancy

Brief to the doctor

Mrs PB is a 34 year old woman who presents with a positive pregnancy test. She wants to know about maternity benefits.

Patient summary

Name	PB
Date of birth (Age)	34
Past medical history	6 week postnatal check completed (19 February) Vaginal delivery with episiotomy (10 January)
Current medication	Diclofenac 50 mg thrice daily x 42T (10 January)

Blood tests   Tests were done 3 weeks ago

Hb	11.2 g/dl (12–15)
MCV	99 (83–105)
White cell count	7.32 (4–11)
Differential count	no abnormalities
Platelet count	354 (150–400)

Tasks for the doctor

Read the NICE guidance on antenatal care, see:
www.nice.org.uk/guidance/index.jsp?action=byIDando=11947

NICE advises that a pregnant woman, at the first contact with a healthcare professional, receives:
- folic acid supplementation
- advice on food hygiene, including how to reduce the risk of a food-acquired infection
- lifestyle advice, including smoking cessation, and the implications of recreational drug use and alcohol consumption in pregnancy
- advice on all antenatal screening, including screening for haemoglobinopathies, the anomaly scan and screening for Down syndrome, as well as risks and benefits of the screening tests

Read guidance on Statutory Maternity Allowance (SMA), see:
www.dwp.gov.uk/lifeevent/benefits/statutory_maternity_pay.asp.

SMA is paid for 39 weeks. In this case, the doctor needs to ascertain when the current maternity leave started and count 39 weeks to determine when it runs out. The case was written for maternity leave to have started on 2 January. Therefore, SMA ends in October.

The earliest date that new SMA can start is from the 11th week before the week the baby is due. In this case, if the EDD for the current pregnancy is 5 November, then SMA may start at the end of August. The patient can be advised to start her new SMA when her current SMA ends.

www.dwp.gov.uk/advisers/ni17a/smp/smp_2.asp:
To qualify for SMA, the patient must be in continuous employment, usually employment by the same employer without a break, except under some circumstances when employment can be treated as continuous in spite of some breaks, such as absence (for periods of 26 consecutive weeks or less) because of sickness, injury, pregnancy or childbirth.

Having read the above guidance, watch case 8 on the DVD. Mark the candidate according to the schedule listed below.

Generic indicators for targeted assessment domains	Descriptors – positive and negative
A. Data gathering, technical and assessment skills • Gathering of data for clinical judgment, choice of examination, investigations and their interpretations • Demonstrating proficiency in performing physical examinations and using diagnostic and therapeutic instruments Maps on the blueprint to: • **Data gathering and interpretation (A)** • **Technical skills (F)**	Positive indicators: • correctly establishes the EDD • takes a focussed obstetric history, establishing the need for folic acid supplementation and iron treatment • elicits what the patient already knows about antenatal care and screening • finds out when current maternity leave commenced, or signposts to resources with information on SMA Negative indicators: • is unable to calculate the EDD • does not identify need for folic acid and iron treatment • appears disorganised or unsystematic in taking a relevant gynaecological and obstetric history • fails to identify when current SMA ends and date from which new SMA can be claimed, or fails to signpost to resources to provide this information

B. Clinical management skills	Positive indicators:
• Recognition and management of common medical conditions in primary care. Demonstrates flexible and structured approach to decision making. • Demonstrating ability to deal with multiple complaints and co-morbidity and to promote a shared approach to managing problems Maps on the blueprint to: • **Management (B)** • **Co-morbidity and health promotion (C)**	• clarifies for patient the date of expected delivery and end of first trimester • discusses routine ANC • prescribes the correct dose of folic acid and ferrous sulphate and takes steps to improve concordance • refers appropriately to the midwife Negative indicators: • fails to clarify for patient the date of expected delivery and end of first trimester • fails to discuss routine ANC • fails to prescribe the correct dose of folic acid and ferrous sulphate and/or fails to improve concordance • fails to refer to the midwife or refers inappropriately to resources for high-risk pregnancies
C. Interpersonal skills	Positive indicators:
• Use of recognised communication techniques that enhance understanding of a patient's illness and promote a shared approach to managing problems • Practising ethically with respect for equality and diversity in line with accepted codes of professional conduct Maps on the blueprint to: • **Person-centred approach (D)** • **Professional attitude (E)**	• shows empathy to the patient's embarrassment and takes steps to put her at ease • involves the patient in the management plan • addresses the patient's expectations regarding SMA and her queries regarding what she should tell her employers Negative indicators: • fails to put the patient at ease or embarrasses her further • fails to involve the patient in the management plan; gives formulaic ANC advice and prescriptions • fails to acknowledge the patient's expectations regarding SMA and employment

Debrief

- What could you learn from this consultation? How to:
  - establish rapport, show empathy and put the patient at ease
  - explore the patient's health understanding regarding ANC so as not to repeat advice
  - take steps to enhance concordance
  - be efficient with time
- How would you focus and structure the history taking?
- What ANC advice would you provide?
- What prescriptions would you write?
- How would you deal with the request for information on SMA and returning to work?

Relevant literature

www.nice.org.uk/guidance/index.jsp?action=byIDando=11947

For information on SMA, see
www.dwp.gov.uk/lifeevent/benefits/statutory_maternity_pay.asp

Video 9 – Pre-wedding diet pills

Brief to the doctor

Miss LA is a 28 year old woman who presents with an internet printout on a 'diet patch.' She wants to know about the efficacy and safety of the patch.

Patient summary

Name   LA

Date of birth (Age)   28

Past medical history   Low back pain (2 months ago) – referred to
                                 physiotherapy

Current medication   Ibuprofen 400 mg thrice daily x 84T (2 months ago)

Tasks for the doctor

This case is written to test how well the candidate consults with a woman presenting with an internet printout. The case is weighted to assess the doctor's interpersonal skills, that is, his ability to consult in a patient-centred manner.

Read the information provided on the advantages and disadvantages of internet printouts, guidance on how to deal with the situation and the characteristics of patient-centred consulting. Then watch the DVD and mark the case.

For information on the pros and cons of internet printouts, see: www.jmir.org/2002/1/e5/. Poor quality information may result in misdiagnosis and mistreatment. However, the advantages are:
- increased information – with improved understanding and self-care
- reduction in clinician consultations
- prompt help-seeking when needed
- a medium for social support, by providing patients with narratives about another's experience of illness. Texts written by patients may provide the personal experience and reassurance desired.

For guidance on how to deal with the internet printouts, see Brown (2003) article in *Pulse*. When a patient presents with an internet printout, try to determine the patient's agenda.
- Why did they do this? What specific questions did they have?
- Are they unhappy with their current management?

- Did they find this exercise useful? If so why?
- Have they had previous experience with online searching?

What should the doctor do?
- Remember patients are asking for the doctor's advice and opinion, probably because they value it.
- Once doctors have elucidated the patient's concerns, questions and anxieties, appraise the information.
- Cross-check with reference sources such as textbooks.
- Discuss the findings.

For the characteristics of patient-centred consulting, see Little *et al.* (2001) in the *BMJ*. Patient-centred care is care which:
- explores the patient's main reason for the visit, concerns, and need for information
- seeks an integrated understanding of the patient's world – that is, their whole person, emotional needs, and life issues
- finds common ground on what the problem is and mutually agrees on management; enhances prevention and health promotion
- enhances the continuing relationship between the patient and the doctor

Having read the above guidance, watch case 9 on the DVD. Mark the candidate according to the schedule listed below.

Generic indicators for targeted assessment domains	Descriptors – positive and negative
A. Data gathering, technical and assessment skills • Gathering of data for clinical judgment, choice of examination, investigations and their interpretations • Demonstrating proficiency in performing physical examinations and using diagnostic and therapeutic instruments Maps on the blueprint to: • **Data gathering and interpretation (A)** • **Technical skills (F)**	Positive indicators: • correctly establishes why the patient presents – for help in appraising the safety and efficacy of the diet patch • elicits why the patient looked for information on the internet • uncovers the patient's concern about her appearance in her wedding dress and in swimwear • finds out what measures the patient has already tried and whether these have been successful Negative indicators: • is bewildered by the information presented; assumes the patient is requesting prescription diet pills • does not identify the patient's wants and needs • does not identify the patient's ideas (herbal is safe), concerns (fat tummy) and expectations (lose 4 lbs in 4 weeks) • makes assumptions about her exercise or diet

B. Clinical management skills	Positive indicators:
• Recognition and management of common medical conditions in primary care. Demonstrates flexible and structured approach to decision making • Demonstrating ability to deal with multiple complaints and co-morbidity and to promote a shared approach to managing problems Maps on the blueprint to: • **Management (B)** • **Co-morbidity and health promotion (C)**	• clarifies for patient that 'herbal' is not synonymous with 'safe' • discusses options for weight loss and sets realistic goals • encourages and supports healthy and sustainable lifestyle changes • promotes a therapeutic relationship and safety-nets Negative indicators: • fails to address safety and efficacy issues • is prescriptive or sets unrealistic goals • prescribes or refers inappropriately • fails to promote the doctor–patient relationship and discourages further consultations
C. Interpersonal skills	Positive indicators:
• Use of recognised communication techniques that enhance understanding of a patient's illness and promote a shared approach to managing problems • Practising ethically with respect for equality and diversity in line with accepted codes of professional conduct Maps on the blueprint to: • **Person-centred approach (D)** • **Professional attitude (E)**	• is sensitive but thorough in exploring the patient's ideas, concerns and expectations • understands the whole person not just her social anxiety • forms a shared understanding with the patient regarding her perception of herself • provides ongoing health promotion – encourages a healthy lifestyle • promotes a therapeutic relationship – is welcoming, facilitative and empowering Negative indicators: • is insensitive, rude or patronising • runs through the 'obesity management' protocol • does not achieve 'shared understanding' – there is a discrepancy between doctor and patient agendas • promotes 'quick fix' measures • promotes excessive reliance on the doctor or inappropriately discourages further consultations

Debrief

- What could you learn from this consultation? How to:
  - establish rapport, by showing a genuine interest in the patient's life within 30 seconds of meeting
  - invite the patient to tell her story – being facilitative and open
  - acknowledge the reason for her attendance, so that she knows you know why she is attending
  - identify her specific concerns and clarify her expectations
  - wind down the discussion, with sentences such as *"how do you feel about it now?"*
- What questions would you ask to 'understand the whole person, not the disease'?
- How would you phrase your health promotion advice?
- How would you develop a therapeutic doctor–patient relationship?

Relevant literature

For information on internet printouts, see:
www.jmir.org/2002/1/e5/

Brown H (2003) Patient with bundle of printouts from the internet. *Pulse*, 24 Nov:
www.pulsetoday.co.uk/story.asp?sectioncode=19&storycode=4002739

Little P, Everitt H, Williamson I, *et al.* (2001) Preferences of patients for patient centred approach to consultation in primary care: observational study. *BMJ,* **322**: 468–472:
www.bmj.com/cgi/reprint/322/7284/468

Potts HW, Wyatt JC (2002) Survey of doctors' experience of patients using the internet. *J Med Internet Res*, **4**(1): e5.
www.bmj.com/cgi/reprint/321/7254/165

Video 10 – Hypnotherapy

Brief to the doctor

Mrs KJ is a 41 year old woman who requests hypnotherapy. She used to see Dr Brown, now retired, for hypnotherapy.

Patient summary

Name	KJ
Date of birth (Age)	41
Past medical history	Contraception (4 months ago)
	Acute on chronic low back pain (6 months ago)
	CT head – no acute changes (14 months ago)
	Severe head injury with frontal lobe damage (18 years ago)
Repeat medication	Microgynon once daily × 126T (4 months ago)

Tasks for the doctor

This case is written to test how the candidate deals with a request for treatment that is not available on the NHS. The case is weighted to assess the doctor's interpersonal skills, that is, his ability to 'give bad news' and deal with the patient's emotions.

Although the framework for 'breaking bad news' has historically been used in consultations communicating the poor prognosis of an illness, the framework can be adapted to consultations in which the patient is given news they do not want to hear, such as the unavailability of certain treatments on the NHS.

Read the guidance on how to communicate bad news and a brief overview of hypnotherapy. Then watch the DVD and mark the case.

For information on how to break bad news, see Faulkner (1998).
- Give bad news in a sensitive manner and at the individual's pace.
- Allow some time before attempting to explore feelings and identify concerns.
- Discuss issues honestly. This may reassure the patient; help him to plan; readjust his hopes and aims.
- Check the reason for the requests directed to you, for example, *"Why the request for hypnotherapy?"*
- Show interest in patient's ideas, for example, *"I wonder if you'd considered any other treatments?"*

- Confirm or elaborate – for example, *"what do you mean by 'a wreck'?"*
- Acknowledge and legitimise the emotion, show concern and remain calm. Displays of emotion from the patient should not be seen as a personal attack.

For information on hypnotherapy, see www.mercurysky.co.uk/bsmdh/faq.htm.
- In therapy, the client relaxes deeply, his attention narrows down, and he focuses on suggestions made by the therapist.
- The suggestions may be aimed at helping the person change the way he responds to a situation, for example, he may be asked to visualise himself taking deep breaths and feeling calm in a confined space.
- Self-hypnotic suggestions may help control anxiety and stress by building self-confidence.
- If a patient lives within the catchment area of a NHS doctor who uses hypnosis, then treatment on the NHS is possible.

Having read the above guidance, watch case 10 on the DVD. Mark the candidate according to the schedule listed below.

Generic indicators for targeted assessment domains	Descriptors – positive and negative
A. Data gathering, technical and assessment skills • Gathering of data for clinical judgment, choice of examination, investigations and their interpretations • Demonstrating proficiency in performing physical examinations and using diagnostic and therapeutic instruments Maps on the blueprint to: • **Data gathering and interpretation (A)** • **Technical skills (F)**	Positive indicators: • explores the reasons for the patient's request • elicits the patient's ideas (she prefers hypnotherapy to anxiolytics for CT scans), concerns (who is going to do the hypnotherapy) and expectations (help in finding a hypnotherapist) • finds out how the problem affects the patient socially – effect on work and relationships • explores the patient's willingness to try alternatives therapies Negative indicators: • does not allow the patient to express their fears about having a CT scan • does not identify the patient's health beliefs • does not identify the psycho-social impact of the patient's anxiety • does not explore options in a way that moves the consultation forward, for example, says *"I'll check and get back to you"*

B. Clinical management skills	Positive indicators:
• Recognition and management of common medical conditions in primary care. Demonstrates flexible and structured approach to decision making. • Demonstrating ability to deal with multiple complaints and co-morbidity and to promote a shared approach to managing problems Maps on the blueprint to: • **Management (B)** • **Co-morbidity and health promotion (C)**	• clarifies for patient that he cannot arrange NHS hypnotherapy • helps the patient plan • shows interest in the patient's ideas, thereby empowering the patient and promoting a therapeutic relationship Negative indicators: • fails to tackle the issue or delays giving the 'bad' news • does not explore solutions to the problem • dismisses the patient's ideas and/or prescribes or refers inappropriately • fails to build a cordial and therapeutic doctor–patient relationship
C. Interpersonal skills	Positive indicators:
• Use of recognised communication techniques that enhances understanding of a patient's illness and promotes a shared approach to managing problems • Practising ethically with respect for equality and diversity in line with accepted codes of professional conduct Maps on the blueprint to: • **Person-centred approach (D)** • **Professional attitude (E)**	• appears sensitive and is led by the patient, that is, information is dripped according to the patient's readiness • seems honest and empathetic • shows genuine concern for the patient's well-being • behaves professionally • appears facilitative, empowering and supportive Negative indicators: • appears blunt, callous or put-upon • appears dishonest or untactful • acts in an uncaring or unconcerned manner • displays impatience, awkwardness or anger • seems dismissive or unwelcoming

Debrief

- What could you learn from this consultation? How to:
  - 'drip' information at the patient's pace
  - facilitate an expression of emotion – use open questions and reflective statements
  - listen actively and respond warmly, demonstrating concern for the patient
  - be professional, courteous and calm when confronted with the patient's emotion
  - be honest about the lack of resources
  - provide on-going support and follow-up, if required
- How would you assess the patient's pace?
- What questions would you ask to uncover the patient's emotions?
- How would you say no, for example, when asked for aesthetic plastic surgery or osteopathy on the NHS?
- How would you demonstrate support to the patient having just informed them that they could not have a particular treatment?

Relevant literature

Faulkner A (1998) ABC of palliative care: Communication with patients, families, and other professionals, *BMJ*; **316**: 130–132, see: www.bmj.com/cgi/content/full/316/7125/130.

For a case study on hypnotherapy for anxiety, see: www.hypnos.co.uk/hypnomag/howard2.htm.

Video 11 – Diarrhoea

Brief to the doctor

Miss TD is a 20 year old woman who presents with diarrhoea.

Patient summary

Name	TD
Date of birth (Age)	20
Past medical history	Chest infection (1 week ago)
	Contraception (3 months ago)
Medication	Amoxicillin 250 mg thrice daily x 15T
	Yasmin once daily x 126T (3 months ago)

Tasks for the doctor

This case is written to test how the candidate deals with a common presentation in general practice. The case assesses the doctor's ability to deal with the clinical problem (diarrhoea) and the subsidiary concerns, namely, occupational and family planning issues.

Read the guidance on how to assess antibiotic-associated diarrhoea, manage gastroenteritis and advise on contraception. Then watch the DVD and mark the case.

For information on how to assess antibiotic-associated diarrhoea, see:
www.emedicine.com/MED/topic3412.htm
- *Clostridium difficile* (CD) produces spores which, when ingested into a human gut, develop into mature bacteria. Antibiotics, by killing off gut commensals, allow the number of CD to increase and this causes problems. CD produce toxins, which cause inflammation, mainly to the large bowel.
- Most cases occur in hospitalised patients.
- Symptoms include mild or moderate watery diarrhoea, crampy abdominal pain, nausea and fever.
- Symptoms start within a few days of starting the antibiotic. However, in some cases symptoms develop up to 10 weeks after finishing a course of antibiotics.
- In mild or moderate diarrhoea, stopping the antibiotic may be the only treatment needed.

For information on managing gastroenteritis, see www.cks.library.nhs.uk/gastroenteritis.

- Red flags in a healthy adult are diarrhoea lasting for more than a fortnight, bloody diarrhoea, pyrexia or recent foreign travel.
- Examine for dehydration, appendicitis and acute abdomen.
- Food handlers, who handle unwrapped or raw food, must be clear of symptoms for at least 48 hours before returning to work.

For information on contraception, see the Faculty of Family Planning guidance. The general advice for women using combined oral contraception who have persistent vomiting or severe diarrhoea for more than 24 hours is to follow the instructions for missed pills (see the 'missed pills' flowchart on page 10 of: www.ffprhc.org.uk/admin/uploads/FirstPrescCombOralContJan06.pdf).

Having read the above guidance, watch case 11 on the DVD. Mark the candidate according to the schedule listed below.

Generic indicators for targeted assessment domains	Descriptors – positive and negative
A. Data gathering, technical and assessment skills • Gathering of data for clinical judgment, choice of examination, investigations and their interpretations • Demonstrating proficiency in performing physical examinations and using diagnostic and therapeutic instruments Maps on the blueprint to: • **Data gathering and interpretation (A)** • **Technical skills (F)**	Positive indicators: • explores the patient's health beliefs, that is, what the patient thinks is causing the diarrhoea • excludes 'red flags' • elicits the patient's concerns (regarding her fitness to handle food and be well for her holiday) • performs a targeted abdominal examination and correctly interprets findings Negative indicators: • does not explore the patient's belief that her antibiotics have caused the diarrhoea • does not exclude red flags • does not elicit the patients concerns • does not perform a targeted examination and/or is incorrect in interpretation of the findings

B. Clinical management skills • Recognition and management of common medical conditions in primary care. Demonstrates flexible and structured approach to decision making. • Demonstrating ability to deal with multiple complaints and co-morbidity and to promote a shared approach to managing problems Maps on the blueprint to: • **Management (B)** • **Co-morbidity and health promotion (C)**	Positive indicators: • explains the diagnosis in appropriate language • the explanation incorporates the patient's health beliefs • involves the patient in the management plan • management is evidence-based Negative indicators: • fails to explain the diagnosis or uses jargon the patient is unlikely to understand • the patient's health beliefs are not addressed • the patient is not given an opportunity to be involved in the management plan • management is not appropriate for the working diagnosis or not in line with current accepted UK general practice
C. Interpersonal skills • Use of recognised communication techniques that enhances understanding of a patient's illness and promotes a shared approach to managing problems • Practising ethically with respect for equality and diversity in line with accepted codes of professional conduct Maps on the blueprint to: • **Person-centred approach (D)** • **Professional attitude (E)**	Positive indicators: • appears empathetic to the patient's condition • shows interest in understanding the patient's concerns – is holistic • if medication is prescribed, the patient is correctly advised on how to take the medication • ascertains whether the patient's concerns and queries were addressed Negative indicators: • appears insensitive or uncaring about the patient's condition • appears disinterested or dismissive of the patient's agenda • if medication is prescribed, the patient is not advised or is incorrectly advised on how to take the medication • fails to confirm mutual agreement

Debrief

- What could you learn from this consultation? How to:
  - explore the patient's ideas, concerns and expectations
  - systematically explore 'red flags'
  - target the examination and relay findings in appropriate language
  - construct a management plan in line with current accepted UK practice
  - appropriately address occupational issues
  - make effective use of resources (time and investigations)
- What would you examine for? Are you able to perform the examination slickly?
- How would you address the patient's health beliefs in your explanation?
- How would you deal with the patient's request for antibiotics, or a sick note?
- How would you encourage concordance?

Relevant literature

For information on gastroenteritis, see:
www.cks.library.nhs.uk/gastroenteritis.

For information on antibiotic-associated diarrhoea (*Clostridium difficile*), see:
www.emedicine.com/MED/topic3412.htm.

For guidance on management of infections in primary care, see:
www.hpa.org.uk/web/HPAwebFile/HPAweb_C/1194947340160.

For an excellent website detailing the examination of the abdomen, see:
http://meded.ucsd.edu/clinicalmed/abdomen.htm#Topical.

Video 12 - Febrile convulsion

Brief to the doctor

Mrs BC is a 35 year old woman who presents for information about her daughter Millie's condition. Millie is 9 months old.

Patient summary

Name	Millie C
Date of birth (Age)	9 months
Past medical history	Up to date with childhood immunisations Normal development to date
Repeat medication	None recorded

Tasks for the doctor

This case is written to test how the candidate deals with an anxious mum who is seeking reassurance and further information about her daughter's prognosis. The case assesses the doctor's ability to discuss risk or likelihood of recurrence and allay maternal anxiety.

Read the guidance on how to assess childhood seizures and reassure effectively. Then watch the DVD and mark the case.

For information on febrile seizures, see Offringa and Moyer (2001).
- A febrile convulsion is a seizure occurring in a child aged 6 months to 5 years, associated with fever arising from infection or inflammation outside the central nervous system in a child who is otherwise neurologically normal.
- 90% occur between 6 months and 3 years.
- The four most common causes are viral infections, otitis media, tonsillitis, and urinary tract infections.
- Current UK practice for the management of febrile seizures include paracetamol, ibuprofen, tepid sponging. Advise parents not to force anything into the mouth when the child is fitting.
- Refer children under 18 months, those with features of meningitis, multiple fits, prolonged fits lasting longer than 15 minutes, systemically unwell children and where parents are anxious or unable to cope.
- Only 1% of children who have had a febrile convulsion go on to develop epilepsy compared with 0.4% who have not.
- The risk of recurrence with simple febrile seizures is 10%.

For information on reassuring patients, see Donovan and Blake (2000).

- Reassurance is an important part of consultations, whether the diagnosis is clear or uncertain.
- Clinicians assume that patients are reassured by clear and confident statements about the diagnosis or the failure to find disease, with patients who remain anxious after such reassurance at risk of being labelled as neurotic or having abnormal illness behaviour.
- Clinicians try, ineffectively, to reduce anxiety by emphasising the mildness, early stage, or non-seriousness of the disorder and the likelihood that patients would recover.
- Effective reassurance acknowledges the patients' problems and incorporates their health beliefs. For examples of explanations patients found reassuring, consult the original article.

Having read the above guidance, watch case 12 on the DVD. Mark the candidate according to the schedule listed below.

Generic indicators for targeted assessment domains	Descriptors – positive and negative
A. Data gathering, technical and assessment skills • Gathering of data for clinical judgment, choice of examination, investigations and their interpretations • Demonstrating proficiency in performing physical examinations and using diagnostic and therapeutic instruments Maps on the blueprint to: • **Data gathering and interpretation (A)** • **Technical skills (F)**	Positive indicators: • encourages mum to provide an account of what happened • obtains sufficient information about the seizure and hospital treatment to exclude need for review, re-examination or referral of Millie • obtains the relevant social information to place the complaint in context Negative indicators: • does not encourage the mum to tell her story – is dismissive, interrupts, or discourages the flow of the story • does not obtain information to exclude need for review, re-examination or referral of Millie – assumes that Millie has been treated appropriately and is fine • does not obtain the relevant social information to place the complaint in context – does not obtain the information about mum's brother

B. Clinical management skills	Positive indicators:
• Recognition and management of common medical conditions in primary care. Demonstrates flexible and structured approach to decision making. • Demonstrating ability to deal with multiple complaints and co-morbidity and to promote a shared approach to managing problems Maps on the blueprint to: • **Management (B)** • **Co-morbidity and health promotion (C)**	• explains the diagnosis in appropriate language – clarifies what a febrile seizure is • the explanation builds on the patient's health belief that different illness can cause fever • involves mum in the management plan – mum is given a clear outline of what to do in future febrile illnesses • management is evidence-based – appropriate antipyretics are advised Negative indicators: • fails to explain the diagnosis or uses jargon mum is unlikely to understand • the explanation does not incorporate mum's health belief • mum is not given an opportunity to be involved in the management plan – mum is simply advised to consult again if Millie is ill without any advice on practical measures she could take before consulting • management is not appropriate for the working diagnosis or not in line with current accepted UK general practice
C. Interpersonal skills	Positive indicators:
• Use of recognised communication techniques that enhances understanding of a patient's illness and promotes a shared approach to managing problems • Practising ethically with respect for equality and diversity in line with accepted codes of professional conduct Maps on the blueprint to: • **Person-centred approach (D)** • **Professional attitude (E)**	• identified and addressed the mum's concerns about risk of recurrence and risk of epilepsy • identified and addressed the mum's expectation for advice on what to do if a 2nd seizure occurs • appears empathetic and interested; is reassuring • ascertains whether mum's concerns and queries were addressed Negative indicators: • does not identify and/or does not address the mum's concerns about risk of recurrence and risk of epilepsy – is dismissive of concerns or implies that the hospital should have provided this information • does not identify and/or does not address the mum's expectation for advice on what to do if a 2nd seizure occurs • appears dismissive or disinterested; does not reassure mum or increase her confidence • terminates the consultation without confirming satisfaction with the discussion or understanding of the information given

Debrief

- What could you learn from this consultation? How to:
  - encourage the patient, verbally and non-verbally, to tell the story
  - negotiate the agenda: *"there are two issues here: firstly, what happened last night and secondly, your concerns about recurrence"*
  - screen for information to exclude the need for review, re-examination or referral
  - assess the patient's starting point – *"You are an experienced mum. How would you..."*
  - acknowledge the patient's feelings and reassure effectively
  - elicit mum's reactions and feelings to the information given
  - check with the mum to see that plans have been accepted and concerns addressed
  - make effective use of resources (time and investigations)
- Review the DVD, particularly mum's description of the seizure, to identify statements that are unclear. How would you clarify these statements?
- How could you periodically summarise to verify your understanding of what mum has said?
- How would you express concern, understanding and a willingness to help?
- How would you encourage mum's contribution to the management plan?
- How would you close the session?

Relevant literature

For information on febrile seizures, see:
Offringa M and Moyer VA (2001) Evidence based paediatrics: Evidence based management of seizures associated with fever. *BMJ*, **323**: 1111–1114:
www.bmj.com/cgi/content/full/323/7321/1111

http://cks.library.nhs.uk/febrile_seizure/management/detailed_answers/
assessing_a_child_who_has_had_a_febrile_seizure#

For information on medical reassurance, see:
Donovan JL and Blake RB (2000) Qualitative study of interpretation of reassurance among patients attending rheumatology clinics: *"just a touch of arthritis, doctor?"*
BMJ, **320**: 541–544:
www.bmj.com/cgi/content/full/320/7234/541

Edwards A, Elwyn G, and Mulley A (2002) Explaining risks: turning numerical data into meaningful pictures, *BMJ*, **324**: 827–830:
www.bmj.com/cgi/content/full/324/7341/827

Video 13 - Allergy test

Brief to the doctor

Mr JH is a 23 year old man who requests allergy testing.

Patient summary

Name	JH
Date of birth (Age)	23
Past medical history	Sprained ankle (L) 8 months ago Sprained wrist (R) 3 years ago
Repeat medication	None

Tasks for the doctor

This case is written to test how the candidate deals with a request for treatment that is available on the NHS but may not be clinically indicated for the patient requesting the test. The case is weighted to assess the doctor's interpersonal skills, that is, his ability to analyse need, negotiate with patients and make effective use of resources. Patients often request tests because of perceived needs. Good communicators are able to elicit the reasons for requests and deal with these (usually emotional) issues tactfully.

Read the guidance on how to make effective use of resources and communicate well with emotional issues. Then watch the DVD and mark the case.

For information on how to make effective use of resources, see *Commissioning Report* (Nov 07):

Key issues that need consideration by clinicians when making requests for individual treatments or procedures:
- that a significant clinical need has been identified
- effective benefit has been established
- alternative treatments have been considered
- the safety and efficacy of the product
- proven clinical evidence
- exceptional circumstances
- cost that may be incurred
- risks have been identified

- the issue of informed consent has been addressed
- National Institute of Health and Clinical Effectiveness guidance (NICE)
- local guidance
- in addition to the above, consideration should be given to the likelihood of measurable improvement in the quality of life of the individuals that would be receiving the treatments or procedures
- requests for funding may also be made for treatments or procedures in relation to individual exceptional circumstances on the grounds that their condition is causing psychological ill health and social isolation

Making effective use of resources (RCGP):

The excellent GP	The unacceptable GP
<ul><li>Only prescribes treatments which make an effective contribution to the patient's overall management</li><li>Takes resources into account when choosing between treatments of similar effectiveness</li></ul>	<ul><li>Consistently prescribes unnecessary or ineffective treatments</li><li>Takes no note of resources when choosing between similar treatments</li><li>Refuses to register patients whose treatment may be costly</li></ul>

For information on how to communicate effectively with emotional issues, see Buckman (2002).

The central technique of acknowledging and addressing emotions is straightforward. The empathic response, for example, is a technique that consists of three steps:
1. identifying the emotion
2. identifying the source of the emotion
3. responding in a way that shows you have made the connection between the first two steps

Having read the above guidance, watch case 13 on the DVD. Mark the candidate according to the schedule listed below.

Generic indicators for targeted assessment domains	Descriptors – positive and negative
A. Data gathering, technical and assessment skills • Gathering of data for clinical judgment, choice of examination, investigations and their interpretations • Demonstrating proficiency in performing physical examinations and using diagnostic and therapeutic instruments Maps on the blueprint to: • **Data gathering and interpretation (A)** • **Technical skills (F)**	Positive indicators: • explores the reasons for the patient's request • elicits the patient's ideas (his symptoms are caused by allergies), concerns (his wife wants pets or a baby) and expectations (an NHS allergy test) • finds out how the problem affects the patient socially – effect on work and relationships • obtains sufficient information to exclude a significant allergic reaction or medical problem Negative indicators: • fails to elicit important parts of the history, such as the reason for the request • does not identify the patient's health beliefs • does not place the request in a psychological or social context • does not obtain sufficient information to exclude a significant allergic reaction or medical problem – makes assumptions • undertakes inappropriate or inadequate examinations
B. Clinical management skills • Recognition and management of common medical conditions in primary care. Demonstrates flexible and structured approach to decision making. • Demonstrating ability to deal with multiple complaints and co-morbidity and to promote a shared approach to managing problems Maps on the blueprint to: • **Management (B)** • **Co-morbidity and health promotion (C)**	Positive indicators: • gives information about allergic reactions and testing in assimilable chunks • clarifies for patient that the request for testing depends on clinical need and intended benefit • takes into account 'exceptional' circumstances Negative indicators: • fails to be guided by the patient's response when giving information about allergic reactions and testing • does not explain why the test is not being arranged • undertakes inappropriate investigations • gives treatments that are inconsistent with best practice or evidence

C. Interpersonal skills	Positive indicators:
• Use of recognised communication techniques that enhances understanding of a patient's illness and promotes a shared approach to managing problems • Practising ethically with respect for equality and diversity in line with accepted codes of professional conduct Maps on the blueprint to: • **Person-centred approach (D)** • **Professional attitude (E)**	• demonstrates active listening and appears sensitive • explores important issues using open and closed questioning • seems understanding • encourages the patient's contribution: the patient feels comfortable to ask questions, seek clarification or express doubts • checks with the patient that plans are accepted and concerns addressed Negative indicators: • consistently ignores, interrupts, or contradicts the patient; appears insensitive • is unable to facilitate the patient's response and clarify issues such that important issues are missed • seems unable to discuss sensitive or personal matters; may act uncaring or unconcerned • displays impatience, awkwardness or anger – the patient feels unable to ask questions, seek clarification or express doubts • does not negotiate with the patient or the patient is given little opportunity to be involved in the management plan

Debrief

- What could you learn from this consultation? How to:
  - take time to listen to patients, and allow them to express their own concerns
  - consider relevant psychological and social factors as well as physical ones
  - use clear language appropriate for the patient
  - use investigations when they will help management of the condition – assess clinical need, intended benefit and exceptional circumstances
  - make sound management decisions which are based on good practice and evidence
- How would you facilitate the expression of a patient's concerns or emotions?
- What questions would you ask to uncover the patient's social circumstances or concerns?
- How would you explain to a patient that an MRI scan for mechanical back pain is not currently needed?
- How would you explore the 'exceptional circumstances' in a patient requesting NHS plastic surgery, such as laser treatment for a facial haemangioma?

Relevant literature

For an example of 'An effective use of resources report', see:
Commissioning Report (Nov 07) by Bury NHS PCT: www.burypct.nhs.uk/fileadmin/
user_upload/Publications/PEC_Papers/2007/20071107/AI_2.3_-_EUR_Annual_
Report.pdf

The headings from Good Medical Practice subdivided by the Royal College of General
Practitioners into the characeteristics and behaviours of 'an excellent doctor' and 'an
unacceptable one', see: www.gpcurriculum.co.uk/rcgp/gmpgp.htm

For information on communicating with emotional issues, see:
Buckman R (2002) Communications and emotions, *BMJ*; **325**: 672:
www.bmj.com/cgi/content/full/325/7366/672

Learning consultation skills for COT and CSA

The aim of this section of the book is to encourage readers to practise patient consultations in preparation for COT and CSA. The reader is required to work out the necessary questions and conduct a 'consultation'.

Each of the 20 cases comprises the following sections.
- *'Summary of the patient'*, including any recent test results – the basic background you need.
- *'Tasks for the doctor'* – what you are expected to establish in the consultation.
- *'More about the patient'* – more about the patient's background and presentation; this section can be used by a study partner to allow them to act as the 'patient'.
- *'Approach to be taken'* – this explains what the examiners are assessing with the case and provides a model answer.
- *'Test your theoretical knowledge'* – a short series of single answer multiple choice questions to test how well you understand current clinical practice; answers are provided at the end of the book.
- Each case ends with suggestions for further reading.

There are two ways to use this section of the book.
1. Ideally, you will work through the cases with a study partner, with one of you assuming the role of 'patient' and the other the role of 'doctor'.
    - The 'patient' reads the first two pages of the case, comprising the *Summary of the patient* and *More about the patient* sections – this allows them to understand the expectations of the patient so they can then answer the doctor's questions.
    - The 'doctor' should read only the first page comprising the *Summary of the patient* and should then conduct a consultation with the patient with a view to:
      A. gathering data to get to the nub of the problem
      B. managing the clinical problem
      C. demonstrating their interpersonal skills

2. Working alone, read through the first page and then note down the questions you would wish to ask in the consultation, referring to the *More about the patient* section as necessary. You may wish to use a COT *pro forma* for your answers.

COT *pro forma*[1]

A. Data gathering, examination and clinical assessment skills

1. Define the clinical problem:
- What questions do you ask to clarify why the patient has presented today?
- How would you explore the patient's ideas, concerns, expectations and health beliefs?

2. Perform an appropriate physical or mental examination
- What is the appropriate targeted physical or mental state examination?
- Can you perform the examination slickly and sensitively using appropriate medical equipment?

B. Clinical management skills

3. Make an appropriate working diagnosis
- On the basis of probability, what is your working diagnosis?

4. Explain the problem to the patient using appropriate language
- How would you explain the diagnosis to the patient?
- Is your explanation jargon-free, well organised and logical?
- Does it address the patient's concerns and expectations?

5. Provide holistic care and use resources effectively
- Was your management plan informed by national or local guidelines?
- Have you referred appropriately?

6. Prescribe appropriately
- Have you considered drug interactions or discussed side effects?
- Did you check the patient's understanding of the medication?

7. Specify the conditions and interval for follow-up
- Have you safety netted appropriately?

---

1   Adapted from a COT *pro forma* developed by Dr David Chadwick, Springfield Surgery, Oxfordshire.

C. Interpersonal skills: know and treat this patient

8. Achieve rapport
- Have you demonstrated active listening, sensitivity, and empathy?
- Have you used the patient's ideas and beliefs in explanations?
- Have you addressed the patient's specific concerns and expectations?

9. Give the patient the opportunity to be involved in significant management decisions
- Have you involved the patient in decisions?
- Have you negotiated, offered various treatment options or encouraged autonomy and opinions?

Case 1 – Menopausal symptoms

Brief to the doctor

Mrs JS is a 51 year old woman who presents for treatment of her hot flushes. She used HRT tablets 2 years ago for peri-menopausal flushing and stopped 3 months ago after developing PV bleeding. Her hysteroscopy 1 month ago was negative. Having discontinued with the HRT 3 months ago, the flushes have recurred.

Patient summary

Name	JS
Date of birth (Age)	51
Social and Family History	Married, two children
Past medical history	Hysteroscopy (1 month ago) – no pathology
	Postmenopausal bleeding on HRT (3 months ago)
	Hip pain (1 year ago)
	Menopausal symptoms (flushing) for 2 years
Current medication	Ibuprofen 400 mg prn x 84

Blood tests — Tests were done 1 month ago (pre-hysteroscopy)

Plasma fasting glucose	5 mmol/l (3.65–5.5)
Fasting cholesterol	5 mmol/l
TSH	1.12
Hb	13.2 g/dl (13–17)
MCV	86 (83–105)
BMI	25.6
BP	117/60

Tasks for the doctor

In this case, the tasks are to:
- present Mrs JS with suitable treatment options for her hot flushes
- provide her with sufficient information to make an informed decision
- prescribe appropriately

Brief to the patient – more about the patient

1. Profile:

- Mrs JS a 51 year old woman
- married with 2 children, ages 18 and 15
- a paediatric out-patient nurse
- flushing is becoming a real nuisance: disturbs sleep, embarrasses her when it occurs at work and she feels tired
- she felt well on HRT but really disliked having a hysteroscopy for PMB so, if possible, would prefer not to restart HRT; she's read about soya and yams but is unaware of other treatment options

2. She is seeing the doctor today because:

- she has not had a period or any PV bleeding for 3 months; prior to this, she had withdrawal bleeds on the HRT
- she is not keen on hormone treatments or the Mirena coil; she does not have any other health problems and uses condoms for contraception
- she is now flushing more than three times per day every other day – her sleep is interrupted and she feels tired
- she is worried about her ability to maintain a calm and reassuring demeanour at work (paediatric OPD) if she continues to feel tired and irritable
- she expects the doctor to give her advice about complementary therapies, prescribe something or refer her to the Menopause Clinic – she wants an action plan for this problem and is not happy with a 'wait and see' policy
- she quickly grasps the medical information imparted and nods her head to indicate understanding of the treatment options
- if she feels coerced into choosing one option (such as HRT), she asks for a referral to the Menopause Clinic
- if the doctor laughs at her health beliefs, she challenges him on his views on complementary therapies
- if the doctor offers her SSRIs, at first she seems sceptical and asks if the doctor thinks she is depressed – she accepts this treatment after a discussion on its evidence, efficacy and safety

Approach to be taken

A. Data gathering, examination and clinical assessment skills

1. *Define the clinical problem: clarify why the patient has presented today*
   The doctor:
   - reads the patient summary provided prior to seeing Mrs JS
   - detects Mrs JS's reluctance to restart HRT and her eagerness to explore alternative treatment options for her menopausal flushing
   - asks open questions to explore the frequency, severity, impact of the flushing, and her specific concerns about HRT
   - asks closed questions to ascertain the presence (or absence) of other menopausal symptoms, including periods
   - excludes red flags, such as on-going PMB
   - elicits how the problem affects Mrs JS at work (and at home)
   - discovers Mrs JS's ideas regarding phytoestrogens
   - discovers her concerns about further episodes of PMB on HRT
   - discovers her expectations for further treatment, either conventional or complementary
   - summarises the problem: *"Mrs JS, on stopping your HRT you have experienced flushes that interfere with your ability to work comfortably. You'd prefer not to take HRT and would like me to discuss alternative treatment options with you. Have I understood you correctly?"*

2. *Perform an appropriate physical or mental examination*
   - In this case, neither a formal physical or mental state examination is required.

B. Clinical management skills

3. *Make an appropriate working diagnosis*
   The doctor, based on the history and exclusion of 'red flags', makes a clinically sound working diagnosis – menopausal flushing.

4. *Explain the problem to the patient using appropriate language*
   The doctor:
   - explains that the menopausal flushing is a 'nuisance' problem rather than a 'serious health problem'
   - agrees with Mrs JS that it should be treated to improve her quality of life
   - discusses in jargon-free language the benefits and risks of HRT (IUS + oestrogen only HRT), SSRIs, and phytoestrogens; may briefly mention 2nd and 3rd line alternatives such venlaflexin, gabapentine or clonidine which can be initiated if recommended by the Menopause Clinic
   - provides information in adequate chunks and checks understanding at each step

- uses the patient's ideas: phytoestrogens may be useful; however, there is little clinical evidence regarding their efficacy and safety (see www.rcn.org.uk/__data/assets/pdf_file/0007/78712/003069.pdf)
- addresses the patient's concerns: further PMB on HRT may require investigation to exclude endometrial pathology, hence endometrial protection with an IUS and oestrogen-only HRT or SSRIs may be more acceptable to the patient
- addresses the patient's expectations – provides treatment options

5. *Provide holistic care and use resources effectively*
   The doctor:
   - may use or discuss complementary medicines, such as Red Clover and Black Cahosh
   - may use time as a therapeutic tool: if Mrs JS seems to have difficulty in making a decision regarding which treatment she would prefer, the doctor could offer a leaflet and provide a follow-up appointment
   - offers the treatment options and, if Mrs JS indicates that she would like to get her treatment sorted out today, helps her to choose the most appropriate therapy for her
   - demonstrates practice of evidence-based medicine – he discusses which treatment options have a good evidence base and are proven to be effective
   - is informed by national or local guidelines – www.cks.library.nhs.uk/menopause

6. *Prescribe appropriately*
   The doctor:
   - if prescribing SSRIs, chooses a cost-effective medication
   - prescribes the appropriate dose and number of tablets
   - discusses drug interactions and side effects
   - checks the patient's understanding of the medication

7. *Specify the conditions and interval for follow-up*
   The doctor:
   - safety-nets appropriately – when to consult again and why: *"Is it OK to meet again in a fortnight to check how you are getting on with this tablet? Obviously, if there are problems, I'd like to see you sooner."*

C. Interpersonal skills: know and treat this patient

8. *Achieve rapport*
   The doctor:
   - listens attentively to the patient's request for treatment and her concerns regarding PMB on HRT
   - displays empathy to the adverse effect flushing has on her confidence and comfort at work

- is non-judgemental about the patient's health beliefs regarding complementary therapies
- addresses the patient's specific concerns and expectations, for example, does not spend more time speaking about HRT and breast cancer when this is not the patient's specific concern; addresses her concern about the difficulty in differentiating between significant endometrial pathology and 'nuisance' break-through bleeding on HRT

9. *Give the patient the opportunity to be involved in significant management decisions*
   The doctor:
   - shares a raft of management options and involves the patient in decisions
   - negotiates with the patient which option may be better for her given her specific concern (HRT and BTB)
   - reassures the patient SSRIs are effective in reducing the frequency of flushing and are not, in this instance, being used to treat a psychological problem
   - encourages autonomy and opinions – with regard to complementary therapies, the doctor provides a balanced discussion regarding evidence, cost, etc., but refrains from making derogatory comments if he does not share these health beliefs

Debrief

Discuss how the doctor could, if needed, improve his performance. In particular, assess whether the doctor:

- empathised? If so, how?
- presented the patient with appropriate treatment options?
- explained the risks and benefits of treatments in simple language

If the consultation over-ran:

- how could the history taking be shortened?
- how could the explanations be simplified?
- how could the doctor have expressed empathy and understanding? Comment on the doctor's non-verbal behaviour and his summarising.

Revising data gathering

Are there any existing medical records for the doctor to peruse before the patient consults?

- The doctor was given a patient summary prior to the patient's presentation.

What questions could the doctor ask to discover the patient's ideas, concerns, expectations and health beliefs?

- Ideas: *"I understand that you are not keen to restart HRT. Were there any other treatments you had in mind?"*
- Concerns: *"You don't seem keen on using SSRIs. Are there particular concerns you have about these tablets?"*
- Expectations: *"It seems to me the flushing is really interfering with your work and you want to discuss the risks and benefits of potential treatments. Shall we run through these options?"*
- Health beliefs: *"You know that SSRIs are used to treat depression. What you may not know is that they are also particularly useful in reducing the frequency of menopausal flushing; it is not being used as an antidepressant here. In addition, there is no added risk of BTB with SSRIs, unlike HRT."*

Once the doctor has gathered sufficient information, how could he summarise the problem for the patient?

- *"Mrs JS, you have given me quite a lot of information. I'd like to summarise our discussion back to you so you can correct me if I've left out anything important."*
- *"You suffer from menopausal flushing. You have used HRT in the past but unfortunately developed BTB. You would like treatment of the flushing, but you would prefer to consider options other than HRT. In particular, you'd like to discuss the effectiveness and safety of natural oestrogens."*

Test your theoretical knowledge

For each of the following statements, answer true (T) or false (F).
1. For vasomotor symptoms, consider a 2 week trial of paroxetine (40 mg daily).
2. For vasomotor symptoms, consider a 2 week trial of citalopram (20 mg daily).
3. Venlafaxine 37.5 mg twice a day is licensed for the treatment of menopausal flushing.
4. There is evidence that smoking cigarettes increases the likelihood of flushing.
5. Ginseng, black cohosh, and red clover may be used in women with contraindications to oestrogen (e.g. breast cancer).

Relevant literature

http://cks.library.nhs.uk/menopause/in_depth/management_issues

Case 2 – Neck pain

Brief to the doctor

Mr AB is a 34 year old man who presents to your surgery with a 4 week history of neck pain that is getting progressively worse.

Patient summary

Name	AB
Date of birth (Age)	34
Social and family history	Single Lives with mother
Past medical history	Road traffic accident 17 years ago • Fracture of right femur and tibial plateau • Fracture of left ankle
Current medication	None

Investigations   2 years ago:

BMI	34
BP	135/90
Urine	NAD on Multistix

Tasks for the doctor

In this case, the tasks are to:
- clarify the neck pain symptoms, identify causative factors (occupational history), perform an appropriate examination, formulate a diagnosis, and finally present Mr AB with appropriate management options and agree on a management plan
- undertake opportunistic screening in view of BMI and BP; explore his health beliefs about weight and identify factors that might motivate him to lose weight

Brief to the patient – more about the patient

1. Profile:

- AB is a 34 year old single man
- he works in the accounts department of a local business
- he has been getting neck pain for the past 4 weeks

2. He is seeing the doctor today because:

- the pain is getting worse; it is localised to the right side of his neck at the back and does not radiate and he has no sensory changes or weakness in the arms. The pain gets worse during the day at work. It does not disturb his sleep and is not present on waking. He does not get the pain at weekends, even though he spends a lot of the time looking after his mother who is 'crippled with arthritis'.
- he has started taking ibuprofen and paracetamol at work to ease the pain
- his work is sedentary, checking account details on the computer
- he would like to be referred for physiotherapy as he believes his pain is due to sitting in front of a computer all day; he is happy to be given postural advice or exercises. He does not like taking tablets as he feels they only mask the problem and he is worried that doing so will result in long term damage to his neck.

3. Additional information:

- If the doctor asks specifically:
  - he has been moved to a different area of the office following a restructuring of the company. His new desk is small and the screen is set to one side, so he has to twist to look at it. He has an adjustable chair, but it is broken and the height is no longer adjustable. He is reluctant to make a fuss, because so many people lost their jobs in the restructuring. He would really like a letter from the doctor to give to his occupational health nurse suggesting that his workplace may be contributing to, or even causing, his neck pain.
  - he has no past history of neck or back pain
  - he is worried that arthritis is hereditary and that he is getting arthritis in his neck
- If the doctor asks about his weight:
  - he has put on more weight since last weighed; his mother is also obese, as was his father until he died of a heart attack age 55 years
  - he snores, but has no daytime somnolence
  - he follows no special diet; his mother likes 'good old-fashioned English food'. He buys sandwiches or crisps for lunch and always has sweets and chocolate in his office drawer. He drinks 1–2 cans of beer in the evenings. He despises smoking.

- o he knows he should lose weight, but finds it difficult to motivate himself, or to do it in isolation from his mother – he thinks eating is one of the few pleasures they both enjoy
- o he is concerned about his future health, especially as his father died of heart disease; if the doctor advises him in unambiguous terms that losing weight would benefit his health, he would address the problem
- if the doctor examines him:

System	Findings
General	Central obesity. Waist 40 inches (102 cm) Posture – rounded shoulders, protruding head BMI 36
Cardiovascular	Pulse 78 SR HS 1+2 nil No evidence of cardiomegaly or cardiac decompensation BP 150/94
Endocrine	No evidence of thyroid disease Urine negative for glucose
Cervical spine	Flexion – slightly reduced due to pain Extension – full Side flexion and rotation – slightly reduced to left, full to right Tender C5/6 on the left
Upper limb neurology	No sensory or motor loss Reflexes intact

Approach to be taken

A. Data gathering, examination and clinical assessment skills

1. *Define the clinical problem: clarify why the patient has presented today*
The doctor:
- reads the patient information provided prior to the consultation – notes the past history of lower limb fractures and raised BMI and BP
- asks open questions to explore and clarify:
  - how Mr AB's neck pain affects him at home and at work
  - Mr AB's feelings about his weight and dieting
  - Mr AB's home circumstances
- empathises with Mr AB over work and home situations
- asks closed questions to exclude 'red flag' symptoms regarding his neck, metabolic causes for his obesity, and to assess his CVD risk
- discovers AB's feelings about medication and his fear that arthritis is hereditary
- uses internal summaries for each area to check that he has obtained the correct information

2. *Performs an appropriate physical or mental examination*
- In this case, an examination is appropriate and should include:
  - posture – cervical spine movements and quick upper limb neurology check for sensation; the patient reports no neurological symptoms, so a detailed neurological examination is not necessary
  - cardiovascular – BP and BMI at minimum; calculate CVD risk
- There is probably insufficient time to consider endocrine problems – hypothyroidism, Cushing's, diabetes, etc. These could be deferred to a follow-up appointment as he feels well.
- Explain the purpose of examination in appropriate language.
- The examination addresses the patient's ideas that his work is causing his pain and his concerns that he is developing neck arthritis.

B. Clinical management skills

3. *Make an appropriate working diagnosis*
The doctor:
- integrates information from the past and occupational histories, the pattern of pain, and the examination findings, to make a working diagnoses of postural neck pain
- identifies that Mr AB has an increased CVD risk due to obesity, BP, lack of exercise, and family history

4. *Explain the problem to the patient using appropriate language*
The doctor:
- addresses Mr AB's agenda:
  - neck pain is probably due to the work-station set-up
  - Mr AB's weight and lifestyle are increasing his risk of CVD
- provides information on posture and workplace set-up, CVD, and losing weight
- explains the need to monitor Mr AB's BP and weight, and for him to modify his lifestyle
- uses 'chunking and checking' to ensure accuracy of data collection and to check Mr AB's understanding at various stages throughout the consultation

5. *Provide holistic care and use resources effectively*
The doctor:
- practices evidence-based medicine – NICE obesity guidelines
- discusses the role of the occupational nurse to assess his workplace
- involves other members of the PHCT, such as the Practice Nurse, to give dietary advice and monitor Mr AB's weight and BP
- understands socioeconomic/cultural background – job losses and having to look after his arthritic mother
- demonstrates to Mr AB that the management of his problems share common features such as losing weight and increasing physical activity

6. *Prescribe appropriately*
The doctor:
- is aware of national and local guidelines (NICE guidelines on obesity and hypertension), and so dietary advice but not medication is indicated here
- reassures Mr AB that the use of intermittent ibuprofen and paracetamol is appropriate to help when pain interferes with work. The doctor should check that there are no contraindications to NSAID use such as indigestion and asthma.
- makes appropriate referral to physiotherapy for advice on self-management
- arranges further checks of BP and weight
- arranges dietary advice
- provides a letter for Mr AB's occupational nurse

7. *Specify the conditions and interval for follow-up*
The doctor:
- signposts Mr AB to information on posture and exercise, and weight management and healthy eating
- offers a follow-up appointment to check progress at work
- offers a follow-up appointment with the Practice Nurse to monitor weight and BP
- confirms understanding

C. Interpersonal skills: know and treat this patient

8. *Achieve rapport*
   The doctor:
   - listens attentively to Mr AB's concerns about his work and home situations
   - recognises verbal and non-verbal cues – Mr AB is reluctant to make a fuss at work as he is concerned about his job security
   - places problem in psychosocial context – how it may affect his ability to look after his mother
   - understands his request for physiotherapy and for a letter to his employers
   - discovers patient's health beliefs, e.g. that his workplace is contributing to his symptoms
   - addresses the patient's specific concerns and expectations

9. *Give the patient the opportunity to be involved in significant management decisions*
   The doctor:
   - encourages autonomy and opinions – provides patient with information and a letter to the occupational nurse to enable patient to tackle the cause of his neck pain
   - supports him in caring for his mother and explores whether additional help is required and would be acceptable to them

Debrief

This case could develop in several directions. The presenting complaint, neck pain, is relatively straightforward and the occupational cause should be identified readily. This should leave time to discuss Mr AB's weight problem and risks of CVD. However, there are other issues such as job insecurity and his mother's arthritis and increasing dependence on him that could deflect the doctor from completing the consultation in the available time.

Discuss how the doctor could, if needed, improve his performance. In particular, assess whether the doctor:
- identified that the neck pain was likely to be an occupational problem
- explored a range of management options with Mr AB – self-management exercises, posture advice, occupational nurse referral to name a few
- took the opportunity to talk about Mr AB's weight problem and the long-term effects of this on his health
- explored Mr AB's health beliefs and motivated him to lose weight and become more active
- arranged suitable investigation (work station assessment) and review

Revising data gathering

What questions could the doctor ask to discover the patient's ideas, concerns, expectations and health beliefs?
- Ideas: *"What do you think may have caused the neck pain?"*.
- Concerns: *"Are you concerned about your weight?"*.
- Expectations: *"It seems that your work may be causing your neck pain, shall we talk about how you might be able to improve things there?"*.
- Health beliefs:
  - *"Your father died of a heart attack at quite a young age, are you worried that this might affect you?"*
  - *"You seem reluctant to take tablets for the neck pain, but if the pain is bad and affecting you, they can be useful, as correcting your posture and workplace may take some time to help things."*.

Once the doctor has gathered sufficient information, how could he summarise the problem for the patient?
- *"We have discussed a lot of issues today, and I would like to summarise back to you in case I've left out anything important or got anything wrong"*.
- *"Your neck pain is most likely to be caused by your new work place; we have talked about how you might improve this at work and also about improving your posture. We have agreed that if things get worse, physiotherapy may ease the symptoms, but will not treat the cause, which you seem keen to tackle first"*.

- *"We have discussed your risk of developing CVD given your family history, your increasing weight and BP. We have agreed to arrange some diet advice and support to lose weight and explore ways you can increase your physical activity".*

Test your theoretical knowledge

For each of the following statements, answer true (T) or false (F).

Regarding NICE guidance on management of obesity
1. BMI results should be interpreted with caution as they are not a direct measure of adiposity
2. Some of the following conditions must be met before bariatric surgery can be recommended – BMI >40; all other methods have failed after trials of at least 6 months; and the patient received intensive management in a specialist obesity service
3. Waist circumference gives information on risk of long-term health problems
4. Bioimpedance is recommended as a substitute for BMI because it is a quick and cheap way of accurately assessing adiposity
5. 5–10% weight loss has been shown to produce measurable health outcomes
6. Sibutramine is contraindicated in patients with high or poorly controlled blood pressure

Relevant literature

NICE (Dec 2006), *Obesity: guidance on the prevention, identification, assessment and management of overweight and obesity in adults and children*:
www.nice.org.uk/nicemedia/pdf/word/CG43NICEGuideline.doc

National Obesity Forum, Guidelines on the management of adult obesity and overweight in primary care:
www.nationalobesityforum.org.uk

Case 3 – Childhood eczema

Brief to the doctor

Mrs CC is a 36 year old woman who presents (without her son) asking for a repeat prescription for his eczema. She hands you a list of his medication.

Patient summary

Name	Darius C
Date of birth (Age)	2
Social and Family History	Only child, parents aged 36 and 33
Past medical history	Treated for a 'flare' 4 weeks ago with antibiotics and eumovate Seen in dermatology OPD 9 months ago – atopic eczema
Repeat medication	Doublebase thrice daily Aveeno at night Hydrocortisone as required or once daily for 7 days Oilatum Plus – use daily in bath

Tasks for the doctor

In this case, the tasks are to:
- clarify Mrs CC's concerns regarding her son's treatments
- review Darius' treatments, particularly efficacy and compliance
- prescribe appropriately

Brief to the patient – more about the patient

1. Profile:

- Mrs CC is a 36 year old woman who has returned to work (part-time) as an administrator
- married with 1 child, Darius, who has had eczema since infancy
- Mrs CC is worried about the severity of her son's eczema

2. She is seeing the doctor today because:

- she requires a repeat prescription of his medication
- she needs a set of emollients for nursery
- she recently attended a dinner party where one of the other guests, a health visitor, spoke to her about a new treatment, an 'anti-cancer' cream for eczema and she wants to talk to you about this
- she has not changed Darius' diet – should she?
- her mother-in-law is keen on taking Darius to see a local homeopath
- when asked about her application of the creams, she talks about applying the treatments conscientiously; she is concerned about nursery – they have only used one tube in three weeks and she uses a tube every week

3. Additional information:

- if the doctor discusses tacrolimus or pimecrolimus with her, she says she would like to read up about this before making a decision; she expects the doctor to signpost her to suitable information
- if Mrs CC feels comfortable with you, she volunteers her opinion on homeopathy – 'it is a load of drivel', however she would like your opinion; she also reveals her concern about her mother-in-law's interference, which she perceives as indirect criticism of her child raising

Approach to be taken

A. Data gathering, examination and clinical assessment skills

1. Define the clinical problem: clarify why the patient has presented today
The doctor:
- reads the patient information provided prior to the consultation
- asks open questions to explore how Darius is getting on with his treatment, the bathing and 'creaming' routine, his recovery from his recent flare, and what she thought helped him to improve
- empathises with her comments about how long the routine takes; this 'connection' with Mrs CC allows her to air her concerns regarding her suspicions that the nursery is not applying the emollients as diligently as she does at home
- asks closed questions to clarify details about the current appearance of the skin and which parts of the body are affected
- asks about current infection (weeping, pustules, malaise), facial eczema, sleep disturbance and nursery attendance, i.e. the doctor excludes red flags signalling the need for review or referral
- discovers Mrs CC's idea that homeopathy is 'drivel', her concern about nursery, her expectation for further information about tacrolimus / pimecrolimus and her health belief that diet may be linked to eczema

2. Performs an appropriate physical or mental examination
- In this case, an examination is not required.

B. Clinical management skills

3. Make an appropriate working diagnosis
- The doctor, based on the history, makes a working diagnosis of childhood atopic eczema; Mrs CC tells you that the dermatologists agreed with this diagnosis and initiated the current treatment regime.

4. Explain the problem to the patient using appropriate language
The doctor:
- having quickly established that Mrs CC is sensible and diligent in her application of the creams, addresses her agenda
- prescribes the medication and asks what she intends to do about nursery
- provides some information on the effectiveness of complementary and alternative (CAM) treatments – very little of it has good trial evidence and some may be harmful, for example, some Chinese herbal medicines for eczema have been found to contain dexamethasone
- explains that the health visitor may have been taking about tacrolimus or pimecrolimus; these immune suppressors may be useful for patients with moderate-to-severe disease, however, there is a theoretical increased risk

of developing skin cancer; they should be initiated by dermatologists or GPs with a special interest in dermatology, so it may be useful to discuss at the next OPD appointment

- advises Mrs CC that most children with atopic eczema do not have food allergy, and that exclusion diets rarely help. The importance of having a healthy balanced diet for growth and well-being is discussed.

5. *Provide holistic care and use resources effectively*
The doctor:
- practises evidence-based medicine
- is informed by national or local guidelines
- if Mrs CC is not overly concerned about the side-effects of steroid creams, then the doctor should not waste time addressing this issue – time is better spent addressing her concerns about diet and homeopathy

6. *Prescribe appropriately*
The doctor:
- is aware of national and local guidelines – www.nice.org.uk/nicemedia/pdf/CG057NICEGuideline.doc
- checks the patient's understanding of the medication and the amounts of medication required

7. *Specify the conditions and interval for follow-up*
The doctor:
- signposts Mrs CC to information on tacrolimus or pimecrolimus
- offers a follow-up appointment to discuss any issues arising from her reading; it would be useful to review Darius 'in the flesh' at this appointment to assess whether he meets criteria for initiation of these drugs

C. Interpersonal skills: know and treat this patient

8. *Achieve rapport*
The doctor:
- listens attentively to Mrs CC's concerns about nursery and her mother-in-law
- understands her request for information on alternative treatments
- displays empathy to the time-consuming routine and chronicity of the illness
- is non-judgemental about the patient's ideas on homeopathy and 'anti-cancer' creams
- addresses the patient's specific concerns and expectations

9. *Give the patient the opportunity to be involved in significant management decisions*
The doctor:
- encourages autonomy and opinions – provides her with information so she feels able to tackle treatment issues with nursery and her mother-in-law
- supports and congratulates her in caring for her son

Debrief

Discuss how the doctor could, if needed, improve his performance. In particular, assess whether the doctor:
- established rapport? If so, how?
- addressed Mrs CC's specific concerns? If so, how?
- discussed the evidence base for immune suppressors, exclusion diets and CAM?
- explained the risks and benefits of treatments in simple language

If the consultation over-ran, did the doctor:
- repeat certain questions when taking the history?
- repeat some explanations?
- address issues the patient was not concerned about?

Revising data gathering

- What questions could the doctor ask to discover the patient's ideas, concerns, expectations and health beliefs?
- Ideas: *"I understand that your mother-in-law is keen on homeopathy. What is your view?"*
- Concerns: *"I agree that if applied as prescribed, nursery should have run out of cream much sooner. Are you concerned that they may not be applying the cream as directed?"*
- Expectations: *"It seems to me your recent discussion with the health visitor led to you to think about alternative treatments. I'll quickly outline the risks and benefits of these immune suppressor creams."*
- Health beliefs: *"You suspect that diet and eczema may be linked. Let's talk about this for a moment."*

Test your theoretical knowledge

For each of the following statements, answer true (T) or false (F).
1. A diagnosis of food allergy should be considered in children with atopic eczema who have reacted previously to a food with immediate symptoms.
2. A diagnosis of food allergy should be considered in infants with failure to thrive.
3. If leave-on emollients are prescribed in large quantities (250–500 g weekly), the child should be reviewed.
4. During flares affecting the face and neck, use moderate potency topical steroids for 3–5 days.
5. NICE recommends that health professionals review repeat prescriptions of products for children with atopic eczema at least twice a year.
6. Topical tacrolimus is recommended, within its licensed indications, as an option for the second-line treatment of moderate to severe atopic eczema, in adults and children aged 1 year and older, that has not been controlled by topical corticosteroids.

7. Healthcare professionals should offer a 1-month trial of a non-sedating antihistamine to children with severe atopic eczema.
8. Healthcare professionals should offer a 1-month trial of an age-appropriate sedating antihistamine to children aged 6 months or over during an acute flare of atopic eczema if sleep disturbance has a significant impact on the child or parents or carers.

Relevant literature

www.nice.org.uk/nicemedia/pdf/CG057NICEGuideline.doc

Case 4 – Tennis elbow

Brief to the doctor

Mrs CD is a 28 year old lady who presents with a right tennis elbow.

Patient summary

Name	CD
Date of birth (Age)	28
Social and family history	Married No children No recorded FH of CVD, DM
Past medical history	Seen 4 months ago: *"Repeat COCP. No problems."*
	Seen 3 months ago: *"Persistent headaches – few weeks. Nil specific. Not unwell. Denies any worries. Diagnosis ?cause. Take OTC analgesia if reqd. Suggest watch and wait."*
	Seen 1 month ago: *"Pain Rt shoulder/neck – 2 weeks.No cause identified. Full range of mvmt neck and shoulder. Declined analgesia. Offered physio but declined this as well."*
Current medication	COCP

Investigations	3 months ago	
BP	132/86	
HR	84	
	2 years ago – normal cervical smear	
Smokes	<10/day	

Tasks for the doctor

In this case, the tasks are to:
- assess the severity of Mrs CD's tennis elbow and agree a management plan
- respond to cues about her marriage and sensitively explore her satisfaction with her marriage and how she might try to improve the situation

Brief to the patient – more about the patient

1. Profile:

- Mrs CD is a 28 year old lady who is married to a leading local businessman who is 50 years old; they have a very comfortable lifestyle – large house, expensive cars and holidays
- she gave up her job as an art teacher when she married 4 years ago – she is frustrated that she is no longer working and gave up a profession
- she tries to occupy herself, but finds this difficult. She had to leave a local art group, which she really enjoyed, because her husband became very jealous that she was mixing with like-minded people, some of whom were her age and male. He has enrolled her in the tennis section at the golf club where he is a member and has bought her lessons there. He takes her to the club and plays golf with business acquaintances while she has lessons, then expects her to help entertain his guests over lunch.
- she feels she is used as a glamorous and vivacious 'trophy wife'
- she would like children, but her husband will not consider this as he feels children would distract him from work and prevent him enjoying his current lifestyle

2. She is seeing the doctor today because:

- her right elbow is sore after tennis; she thinks she can probably cope with it, but her husband has insisted she consult, in case it is something serious
- the elbow does not hurt at any other time. Her husband noticed it because she complained that her elbow hurt when driving him home after a business lunch. There has never been any swelling or loss of movement, nor any neurological symptoms. Her neck pain has gone.
- she does not expect or want any treatment. She would be very happy to be told to rest and avoid tennis for a while. She is not at all keen on medicines and prefers to use 'natural' remedies whenever possible.

3. Additional information:

- if the doctor asks specifically:
  - she feels very unhappy with her life and her marriage in particular – she regrets getting married and feels trapped
  - if pressed, she would accept that her presentations with persistent headaches, sore neck/shoulder and elbow pain are reflections of her unhappiness
- she would like the opportunity to talk about how she feels, but only after the doctor has given her enough time and information to enable her to reassure her husband that her elbow pain has been taken seriously. She will not raise

the subject, but will talk freely if the doctor raises the issue. She hopes that by dropping cues that she feels pressured into playing, and that she is not that bothered if told to rest completely, the doctor will suspect there is another matter she wishes to raise. However, if he asks her *"Is there anything else you want to talk about?"* without putting this into context, she will answer *"no"*. She feels that the last doctor that saw her realised there was something else going on, but attempted to 'fob her off' by offering her physiotherapy.

- if asked:
  - she watches her weight very carefully as her husband criticises her if she gains any
  - she has trouble getting to sleep and wakes several times every night
  - she gets tearful easily and tries to avoid talking or thinking about her life because doing so upsets her
  - she has briefly considered suicide but dismissed the idea instantly as she wants to enjoy life not get out of it
  - she feels her parents would be very unsupportive as they disapproved of her marrying someone older and she thinks their attitude would be 'told you so' which she thinks would not be helpful; she is an only child
  - she has no close friends currently; however, she occasionally contacts an old boyfriend who is always very sympathetic and supportive – she occasionally thinks she should have married him
- if the doctor examines her:

System	Findings
Neck	Full range of movement Posture normal
Shoulder	Full range of movement Normal scapulothoracic rhythm
Elbow	Flexion/extension – full and pain-free Pronation/supination – full and pain-free No effusion Very slight tenderness on deep palpation over the lateral epicondyle No pain on resisted wrist dorsiflexion
Forearm	No swelling or tenderness
Neuro	No altered sensation or weakness; reflexes intact Neural tension tests negative

Approach to be taken

A. Data gathering, examination and clinical assessment skills

1. *Define the clinical problem: clarify why the patient has presented today*
   The doctor:
   - reads the patient information provided prior to the consultation, identifying several recent consultations for 'minor' problems
   - asks open questions to explore the presenting reason for her attendance (husband's concern), to clarify her symptoms (minor) and to ascertain how they affect her (minimally)
   - asks closed questions to exclude the neck as a cause of her pain
   - listens attentively and responds to cues such as her feeling pressurised into playing tennis
   - explores whether there are other issues she wishes to discuss using open and closed questions, silence and reference to previous attendances

2. *Performs an appropriate physical or mental examination*
   - In this case, a targeted examination is required – the minimally acceptable examination would be to exclude restricted elbow joint movement (flexion, extension, pronation and supination) and localised swelling or tenderness
   - the examination should address the patient's (and her husband's) concerns
   - a 'gold standard' examination would include neck and shoulder movements and systematic examination of the upper limb

B. Clinical management skills

3. *Make an appropriate working diagnosis*
   The doctor:
   - integrates information from previous consultations, questions about her presenting complaint, cues and questions about her happiness
   - identifies and explores, by using a patient-centred approach, the real reason for the patient's attendance
   - makes a working diagnosis of mild tennis elbow and underlying marital unhappiness

4. *Explain the problem to the patient using appropriate language*
   The doctor:
   - having quickly established that this was a case of mild tennis elbow, gives appropriate management advice – rest from tennis
   - agrees with the patient that medication and referral for physiotherapy are not appropriate
   - provides some information on the effectiveness of complementary and alternative (CAM) treatments – acupuncture/dry needling, and exercises and self-management techniques may help

5. *Provide holistic care and use resources effectively*
   The doctor:
   - does not make an unnecessary physiotherapy referral or prescribe analgesia
   - by exploring the socioeconomic/cultural background, is likely to discover the real reason for the attendance

6. *Prescribe appropriately*
   The doctor:
   - agrees not to prescribe any medication
   - explores a range of management strategies to deal with her unhappiness – how she might raise her frustration at no longer working and having to be a 'trophy wife' with her husband

7. *Specify the conditions and interval for follow-up*
   The doctor:
   - offers a follow-up to explore her feelings about her marriage

C. Interpersonal skills: know and treat this patient

8. *Achieve rapport*
   The doctor:
   - listens attentively to Mrs CD's explanations of her symptoms
   - explores and clarifies her symptoms and feelings
   - recognises verbal and non-verbal cues – not being concerned about having to rest from tennis
   - sensitively explores Mrs CD's unhappiness with her marriage and frustration with her lifestyle
   - places the problem in psychosocial context – her husband pressurising her to play tennis
   - discovers the patient's health beliefs and understands her reluctance to have medication

9. *Give the patient the opportunity to be involved in significant management decisions*
   The doctor:
   - actively confirms patient's understanding of the problem, i.e. that her tennis elbow is mild and requires no active treatment
   - supports and empathises with her marital unhappiness
   - explores various strategies for improving her lifestyle and hence happiness

Debrief

The presenting symptom, tennis elbow, is minor and the real issue in this consultation is picking up the patient's cues about her marriage and then exploring this issue.

Discuss how the doctor could, if needed, improve his performance. In particular, assess how the doctor:
- established rapport with Mrs CD
- identified the underlying issue
- explored strategies Mrs CD might employ to raise or address her unhappiness

Revising data gathering

What questions could the doctor ask to discover the patient's ideas, concerns, expectations and health beliefs?
- Ideas: *"Are you happy that I have excluded a serious problem with your elbow?"*
- Concerns: *"You said that your husband has made you come today, why do you think he has done that?"*
- Expectations: *"It seems to me that the last few times you have come here you have had problems that you didn't want any treatment for. Sometimes that happens when people are worried about something else and so I wonder if there is another problem, perhaps a personal one, that you would like to discuss?"*
- Health beliefs: *"I see you were not keen on painkillers before, is that because you don't like taking medicines?"*

Once the doctor has gathered sufficient information, how could he summarise the problem for the patient?
- *"Your elbow pain does not seem to interfere with you that much and my examination is pretty normal"*

If the consultation over-ran, did the doctor:
- allow the patient to repeat herself or not offer useful information?
- not understand why the patient had attended?
- not pick up the patient's cues?
- find it difficult discussing personal issues and feelings with the patient?
- spend too much time data gathering and not enough time listening?
- fail to organise and structure the consultation appropriately?

Test your theoretical knowledge

For each of the following statements, answer true (T) or false (F).

Regarding tennis elbow
1. It is an overuse injury involving the flexor muscle origin on the lateral epicondylar region of the humerus
2. Pain may radiate into the forearm

3. 90% or more of cases respond to conservative management
4. Corticosteroid injections give rapid and lasting relief
5. Extracorporeal shock wave treatment has been shown to be beneficial
6. Topical nitric oxide (by applying GTN patches) may improve outcome
7. The current fashion for oversized racquets with high string tension increases the risk of developing tennis elbow

Relevant literature

Bisset L, Paungmail A, Vicenzino B, *et al.* (2005) A systematic review and meta-analysis of clinical trials on physical interventions for lateral epicondylalagia. *Br J Sports Med,* **39**: 411–422.

Paoloni JA, Appleyard RC, Nelson J, *et al.* (2003) Topical nitric oxide application in the treatment of chronic extensor tendinosis at the elbow: a randomised, double-blinded, placebo-controlled clinical trial. *Am J Sports Med,* **31**: 915–920.

Smidt N, van der Windt D, Assendelft W, *et al.* (2002) Corticosteroid injections, a physiotherapy, or wait-and-see policy for lateral epicondylitis: a randomised controlled trial. *Lancet,* **359**: 657–662.

Waugh EJ, Jaglal SB, Davis AM (2004) Computer use associated with poor long-term prognosis of conservatively managed lateral epicondylalgia. *J Orthop Sports Phys Ther,* **34**: 770–780.

Case 5 - Ankle injury

Brief to the doctor

Mr TP is a 22 year old man who presents with a sore ankle (right). He walks into your surgery on crutches. He is due to leave for Ghana in 5 weeks as part of a VSO team.

Patient summary

Name	TP
Date of birth (Age)	22
Social and Family History	Unmarried
Past medical history	Tonsillitis 3 years ago Insomnia 6 years ago
Current medication	None
Blood tests	Tests were done 4 months ago (VSO medical)
BMI	27
BP	128/68

Tasks for the doctor

In this case, the tasks are to:
- assess how the ankle injury impacts on his life
- provide him with information about healing times
- help him to reach a decision about physiotherapy and his fitness to undertake volunteer work in a remote area

Brief to the patient – more about the patient

1. Profile:

- Mr TP is a 22 year old man
- unmarried and not currently in a relationship
- works with his father in the building trade undertaking barn conversions and building renovations
- due to start a 3-month VSO placement in Ghana in 5 weeks
- injured his ankle during a football game with his mates 7 days ago; attended A&E where an X-ray ruled out an ankle fracture – he was told to take analgesia and to see his GP for further treatment
- in the week since the injury, he has mobilised well on crutches, is now weight-bearing on the ankle and takes one 400 mg ibuprofen thrice daily

2. He is seeing the doctor today because:

- the A&E doctor told him he didn't have a fracture but didn't give any advice about mobilizing or running
- the box of tablets he was given says he should take one tablet three times a day after meals – for how long should he continue with the tablets?
- he has tried putting weight through the ankle and has walked from his bed to the toilet without crutches – although it was painful (5/10), it was bearable
- what should he do about crutches; when can he start running again; does he need physiotherapy?
- he would like to know if his ankle will be healed within 5 weeks; he is worried about letting his VSO team members down if he needs extra help or if he cannot carry out certain physical tasks such as helping to build a water pipe; also, in Ghana, he will be living in a remote rural area some distance from medical care
- when he contacted VSO for advice, they advised him to consult his GP first
- he does not have private health insurance; if you advise him to pay to see a physiotherapist, he is happy to do so, especially if you think physiotherapy can get his ankle strong again for his Ghana trip
- if the doctor offers him a 'wait and see' policy, he wants to know what he should tell VSO
- if the doctor offers him an NHS physiotherapy referral, he wants to know the likelihood of being seen within 5 weeks
- by the way, he has season tickets to the local football club (worth approximately £550); his parents don't go to games, so would the doctor like the tickets? He is grateful to the practice for organising his VSO medical at short notice and for waiving their fee.

Approach to be taken

A. Data gathering, examination and clinical assessment skills

1. *Define the clinical problem: clarify why the patient has presented today*
   The doctor:
   - notes, from the medical record, that Mr TP had a VSO medical 4 months ago
   - detects a non-verbal cue – Mr TP walks in on crutches; on questioning the reason for the crutches, the doctor obtains a history of the ankle injury and the hospital treatment
   - asks open questions to explore what specifically about the ankle injury brings him to the surgery today, i.e. the doctor explores his expectations and concerns
   - asks focused and closed questions to clarify details of the pain, analgesia, and ability to mobilize
   - elicits how the problem affects Mr TP and discovers his concerns about being fit to travel to Ghana in 5 weeks as part of a VSO team
   - explores his health beliefs that physiotherapy would lead to quicker healing
   - summarises the problem: as regards your ankle sprain, you are consulting today for advice on painkillers, when to restart running, and whether you should go to Ghana in 5 weeks – have I understood you correctly?

2. *Perform an appropriate physical or mental examination*
   - An examination of the ankle is unlikely to be needed given the history of improvements (in pain and mobility) and the fact that the patient does not have specific concerns warranting physical reassessment.

B. Clinical management skills

3. *Make an appropriate working diagnosis*
   The doctor:
   - recognises from the history that the patient is describing a typical grade 2 ankle sprain (www.cks.library.nhs.uk/patient_information_leaflet/sprains)
   - recognises that the ankle injury is healing as it should be (i.e. following the expected pattern of illness)

4. *Explain the problem to the patient using appropriate language*
   The doctor:
   - is patient-centred – uses the patient's ideas on mobilizing (without crutches) as pain allows, reducing NSAIDs and perhaps changing to analgesics, and starting rehabilitation of the ankle (explaining that running may not be the best way to achieve ankle strength and stability – www.cks.library.nhs.uk/sprains_and_strains/in_depth/management_issues)

- uses the patient's beliefs regarding physiotherapy – explains that initial physiotherapy treatment with ultrasound or infrared attempts to reduce swelling and pain, and that later rehabilitation teaches stretching and strengthening exercises to prevent re-injury
- provides information on healing times: grade 2 sprains – people usually start walking on the ankle after 2 days of rest; the swelling goes down after 7–10 days; people in physically demanding jobs may take a few weeks to return to work and people may not be able to take part in sport for a few months
- addresses the patient's concerns and expectations – explores the risks and benefits of postponing the VSO trip until the ankle has regained full strength (this may take a few months) versus going to Ghana where walking on uneven ground may put an incompletely healed ankle at risk of re-injury

5. *Provide holistic care and use resources effectively*
The doctor:
- may, after discussion with the patient, refer to physiotherapy (NHS or private based on his preference)
- practises evidence-based medicine
- is informed by national or local guidelines – www.cks.library.nhs.uk/sprains_and_strains/in_summary

6. *Prescribe appropriately*
The doctor:
- is aware of national and local guidelines
- chooses cost-effective medication (paracetamol rather than codeine; ibuprofen rather than alternative NSAIDs)
- checks the patient's understanding of the medication and warns the patient about potential side effects

7. *Specify the conditions and interval for follow-up*
- The doctor outlines expected healing times and advises the patient to return for re-assessment if he does not heal as predicted

C. Interpersonal skills: know and treat this patient

8. *Achieve rapport*
The doctor:
- understands how important the VSO trip is to him and displays empathy with his bad luck
- addresses the patient's specific concerns (about rehabilitation) and his expectations regarding VSO
- thanks the patient for his offer of the football tickets, which raises an ethical issue: does the offer affect the doctor's decision-making in any way; how does the doctor politely refuse the gift; if the gift is accepted, does the

doctor explain to Mr TP the new stipulation in the GP contract that GPs keep a register of gifts with a value over £100?

9. *Give the patient the opportunity to be involved in significant management decisions*
The doctor:
- shares his thoughts on healing times, the value of rehabilitation and involves the patient in decisions
- encourages autonomy and opinions – asks Mr TP questions that allow him to evaluate the benefits and risks of going to Ghana in 5 weeks, thus facilitating his decision-making

Debrief

Discuss how the doctor could, if needed, improve his performance. In particular, assess whether the doctor:

- understood the reason for the patient's attendance today or whether he made assumptions regarding the patient's agenda? If so, what questions or explanations did the doctor use that led him down this incorrect track?
- asked questions that facilitated Mr TP's decision-making or did the doctor make decisions for him?
- deal with the gift ethically and sensitively?

If the consultation over-ran:
- did the doctor repeat his questions or explanations?
- perform any unnecessary examinations?
- get embarrassed or flummoxed by the gift?

Revising data gathering

What questions could the doctor ask to discover the patient's ideas, concerns, expectations and health beliefs?

- Ideas: *"I understand that you want your ankle to heal as fast as possible. Did you have any ideas on how we could achieve this?"*
- Concerns: *"What is your ankle injury preventing you from doing, at work or socially? Is there anything in particular about your fitness that concerns you?"*
- Expectations: *"When you came into surgery today, what is it that you hoped I would do for you?"*
- Health beliefs: *"Am I right in thinking that you believe the ankle will heal faster with physiotherapy? Let's talk about what improves ankle healing in the short and long term."*

Test your theoretical knowledge

For each of the following statements, answer true (T) or false (F).
1. Rest sprained ankles for 24 hours, after which active movement should be encouraged.
2. Place a bag of ice on to the swollen ankle for 20 minutes, allowing 2 hours in between applications for re-warming.
3. Advise patients to improve balance by walking with the eyes shut, once the pain has settled.
4. Ibuprofen, prescribed to patients with cardiovascular disease, may reduce the cardiovascular protective effect of low-dose aspirin.
5. More than 75% of ankle injuries are ankle fractures.

Relevant literature

www.cks.library.nhs.uk/sprains_and_strains/view_whole_guidance

Case 6 - MRI result - back pain

Brief to the doctor

Mr EF, age 42, wishes to discuss the treatment options for his back following a recent MRI scan organised by the hospital orthopaedic department. He has previously been seeing one of your partners who is now on maternity leave.

Patient summary

Name	EF
Date of birth (Age)	42
Past medical history	1 year ago – GP notes:*"LBP with Rt L5 pain and paraesthesia – 3 months. Private physio and osteopath have not helped. Ibuprofen and Co-codamol 30/500 (prescribed by dental colleague) not helped. V stiff L spine. SLR 30 on Rt, 90 on Lt. Absent Ankle Jerk. Letter from physio suggesting referral. Refer Orthopaedics"*
	9 months ago – Letter from Specialist Physio Clinic: *"5 months LBP with L5 sciatica. No red flags. Has only had manipulative treatment in private sector, for outpatient physio."*
	7 months ago – GP notes: *"Hospital physio referred him for more physio – v unhappy. Getting worse. Interfering with ability to work, considering having to reduce workload, partners at work not happy with him. Wants to see orthopaedic consultant not physio. Letter to consultant requesting he review patient."*
	5 months ago – Consultant letter: *"Thank you for asking me to see Mr EF. I think the time has come to establish the cause of his back and leg pain and have arranged an MRI. I have warned him that there is likely to be a wait for this. I will see him when he has had the scan to discuss treatment options."*
	2 weeks ago – MRI result: *"Reduced signal L4/5 and L5/S1 discs. There is a large Rt sided disc protrusion compressing the L5 root."*

| **Current medication** | Ibuprofen 400 mg 1 tab 3 or 4 times daily with food |
| | Co-codamol 30/500 2 tabs 4 times daily as required |

Tasks for the doctor

In this case, the tasks are to:
- explain the MRI result and treatment options to Mr EF
- explore his concerns about treatments and their long and short-term effects on his health and work (expectations)
- support and explore his disappointment with the quality of care he has received from the hospital

Brief to the patient – more about the patient

1. Profile:

- 42 year old partner in a local private dental practice and is married with 2 children aged 10 and 8 years
- he developed low back pain and right sciatica 15 months ago and initially saw an osteopath and then a physiotherapist privately, but did not respond to treatment. His physiotherapist advised that he needed a scan and possibly an operation. He therefore attended his GP and was referred to the orthopaedic department at the local hospital for an MRI.
- he was seen by a specialist physiotherapist at the hospital who was very critical of the treatment he had received from both the osteopath and from the physiotherapist. He was told there was no indication for an urgent scan and that he should attend the hospital outpatient physiotherapy department for 'proper' physiotherapy.
- he was very unhappy at not being seen by a consultant as he feels that it was discourteous to a fellow health practitioner; he was not happy with the clinic recommendations, but did not want to make a fuss and so complied with the recommendations
- attending physiotherapy outpatients was very disruptive to his practice as the department only offered appointments during the working day. He had already reduced his workload with his partners' agreement, but he sensed that they were getting disgruntled with his reduced presence and contribution to the practice.
- his symptoms did not respond to outpatient physiotherapy and so he saw his GP again and requested a consultant appointment. When he saw the consultant, he was immediately referred for an MRI scan.

2. He is seeing the doctor today because:

- he had the scan 2 weeks ago and would like to know the result
- he has an outpatient appointment in 6 weeks, and would like to discuss what treatments he is likely to be offered by the consultant
- he is concerned that he may never return to full working ability again, even after a back operation
- he wonders whether he would have got better and quicker treatment if he had been seen privately or if he had the MRI earlier
- if there is time, he would like to discuss making a complaint about the treatment he has received at the hospital, particularly the delay in getting the MRI

3. Additional information:

- if the doctor asks specifically:
  - he has constant back and leg pain and is kept awake by pain and so sleeps only fitfully

- o he feels that his right leg is getting weak and the pins and needles are now constant. Coughing, sneezing and straining produce leg pain. He has no problems with bowel or bladder control and no perineal numbness. His weight is stable.
- o his pain is made worse by bending or twisting, which he has to do frequently at work
- o he is a keen runner but has not been able to run since his back pain started
- o the constant pain and lack of sleep are making him grumpy and short-tempered; while he manages to control this at work, if pressed, he has taken it out on his wife and children, but has never been violent.
- he is concerned that his business partners could ask him to leave the partnership or reduce his share of the profits due to his reduced workload. With 2 children at private school, he cannot afford to reduce his income.
- he believes that an operation is indicated and that if the hospital had listened to his GP and private physiotherapist, he could have had the operation by now and hence not be worrying about the effects on work, as well as sparing him and his family from the effects of his worsening symptoms
- he does not want an epidural and will refuse a referral to the Pain Clinic
- he trusts his GPs as they have always given him honest, sensible and unbiased advice
- he does not like to make a fuss and looks to his GP to be his advocate, but feels he should be treated as a priority due to the adverse effect of his problem on work and home
- he has some savings and has discussed with his wife whether to use these to fund an operation privately in order to get it done quickly
- if the doctor examines him:

System	Findings
General	Walks slowly and sits with difficulty Looks tired and drawn
Lumbar spine	Flattened lordosis Flexion-fingertips to top of patella Extension – nil Side flexion – reduced to the right more than to the left Tender palpation L4/5 and L5/S1 Spasm and tenderness of paraspinal muscles
Neurology	SLR 70 left with some cross pain, 20 right Slump test pos. on right Femoral stretch negative bilaterally Absent sensation L5 (right) Weak big toe extension and foot eversion (right) Absent ankle jerk (right)

Approach to be taken

A. Data gathering, examination and clinical assessment skills

1. *Define the clinical problem: clarify why the patient has presented today*
   The doctor:
   - reads the patient information provided prior to the consultation
   - uses a well organised approach to gather information
   - asks open questions to explore how Mr EF is getting on in terms of symptoms and how they are affecting his life – *"How is all this affecting you at work and home?"*
   - asks closed questions to clarify details about level of pain, weakness and paraesthesia, and to exclude cauda equina symptoms
   - discovers Mr EF's belief that an operation is required and that this should be done as soon as possible
   - explores and clarifies the impact his symptoms are having on his home life

2. *Performs an appropriate physical or mental examination*
   - In this case, an examination is required as Mr EF has indicated that his symptoms have worsened, in particular that he has developed weakness.
   - A targeted examination should be made concentrating on lower limb neurology.

B. Clinical management skills

3. *Make an appropriate working diagnosis*
   - The doctor integrates information from the history, scan result and examination, and makes a working diagnosis of L5 nerve root compression due to prolapsed lumbar intervertebral disc.

4. *Explain the problem to the patient using appropriate language*
   The doctor:
   - uses the patient's ideas and beliefs and explains the MRI result and indicates that the consultant is most likely to offer an operation – *"Do you know much about back operations?"*
   - explains the natural history of prolapsed discs
   - outlines the various options available while not pre-empting the consultant's opinion – operation, epidural, pain clinic
   - provides some information on recovery times and functional outcomes from operations in order to address the patient's concerns
   - reviews the effectiveness, or not, of Mr EF's current analgesia
   - checks understanding – *"Does my explanation make sense? Is there anything else you would like to ask?"*

5. *Provide holistic care and use resources effectively*
The doctor:
- practises evidence-based medicine
- is informed by national or local guidelines
- understands and explores the socioeconomic background – effects on work and home life

6. *Prescribe appropriately*
The doctor:
- reviews Mr EF's current analgesia regimen and prescribes tramadol
- checks the patient's understanding of the medication and the amounts of medication required
- discovers whether Mr EF would like to elect for private treatment at this point in time or wait to see the outcome of the outpatient appointment
- decides whether to discuss the urgency of the case with the consultant based on the history and examination findings, but also in view of the patient's dissatisfaction with the treatment received thus far

7. *Specify the conditions and interval for follow-up*
- The doctor ensures Mr EF is aware of the 'red flag symptoms' – safety netting

C. Interpersonal skills: know and treat this patient

8. *Achieve rapport*
The doctor:
- listens attentively to Mr EF's description of his symptoms and their effect on work and home
- may use verbal and non-verbal cues to clarify the degree of Mr EF's disability: "*You seem to have difficulty moving around, is that causing you any problems?*"
- places problem in a psychosocial context – how it affects patient/family
- understands his request for information on recovery and success of treatments
- displays empathy – "*How are you coping?*"
- explores patient's health ideas, concerns and expectations
- is understanding but non-judgemental about the advice and opinion Mr EF was given in his initial hospital appointment; gives advice about making a complaint if Mr EF requests this
- supports Mr EF's efforts to continue working and remain active

9. *Give the patient the opportunity to be involved in significant management decisions*
The doctor:
- actively confirms the patient's understanding of the problem
- shares thoughts/involves patient in deciding how to progress management: "*There are a number of options here... Which of these do you prefer?*"

Debrief

Discuss how the doctor could, if needed, improve his performance. In particular, assess whether the doctor:
- achieved rapport
- dealt with Mr EF's unhappiness with aspects of his treatment by the hospital
- addressed Mr EF's concerns about the impact on his ability to work both in the short and the long term

If the consultation over-ran, did the doctor:
- manage the time available appropriately and in a structured and organised way?
- concentrate on addressing the issues Mr EF was most concerned about (impact on work and family life) or get bogged-down dealing with some aspects of the case (dissatisfaction with the hopsital)?

Revising data gathering

What questions could the doctor ask to discover the patient's ideas, concerns, expectations and health beliefs?
- Ideas: "*Now the scan has confirmed the clinical diagnosis of a disc prolapse, what treatment do you think the consultant is likely to recommend?*".
- Concerns: "*You have told me that you feel under pressure from your partners because you have had to reduce your workload; how do you think they are going to feel if you have to have an operation?*".
- Expectations: "*It seems to me that you believe you need an operation, would you like me to outline the basic options available to you?*".
- Health beliefs: "*You seem concerned that your symptoms may not recover after an operation, would you like to discuss the success rates of operations with myself or the consultant?*".

Test your theoretical knowledge

For each of the following statements, answer true (T) or false (F):
1. The reported lifetime prevalence of back pain varies between 49 and 70%
2. Rare causes of sciatica include tumours and lumbar stenosis
3. Straight leg raising (Lasègue's sign) is a very sensitive and specific test
4. Computed tomography and magnetic resonance imaging are equally accurate at diagnosing lumbar disc herniation
5. Surgical discectomy provides faster relief from acute sciatica than conservative management

Relevant literature

Gibson JN, Waddell G. (2007) Surgical interventions for lumbar disc prolapse. *Cochrane Database Syst Rev,* **1**: CD001350.

Carragee EJ. (2005) The surgical treatment of disc degeneration: is the race not to be too swift? *Spine,* **5**: 587–588.

Koes BW, van Tulder MW, Peul WC. (2007) Diagnosis and treatment of sciatica. *BMJ,* **334:** 1313–1317.

www.lowbackpain.tv

Case 7 - Foot pain

Brief to the doctor

Mr SF is a 37 year old man who presents with a 4-day history of worsening foot pain (right). He requests analgesia. He had blood tests done 5 months ago and was advised to make lifestyle changes.

Patient summary

Name	SF
Date of birth (Age)	37
Social and Family History	Married, two children
	Dad fatal MI aged 69
Past medical history	Hypercholesterolaemia (5 months ago)
	Morton's neuroma 2nd left toe (1 year ago)
	Gout (2 years ago)
Current medication	None

Blood tests — Tests were done 5 months ago

Plasma fasting glucose	5.8 mmol/l (3.65–5.5)
Fasting cholesterol	7.2 mmol/l
Fasting HDL cholesterol	0.8 mmol/l (0.8–1.8)
Total cholesterol:HDL	9
TSH	1.89 (0.35–5.5)
Alkaline phosphatase	156 IU/l (95–280)
Total bilirubin	14 µmol/l (3–17)
Albumin	46 g/l (35–50)
Creatinine level	99 µmol/l (70–150)
BMI	34
BP	141/86
Framingham	12%
Plasma urate (2 years ago)	467 (210–480)

Tasks for the doctor

In this case, the tasks are to:
- advise Mr SF on analgesia and prescribe appropriately
- talk to Mr SF about his lifestyle changes
- arrange suitable follow-up

Brief to the patient - more about the patient

1. Profile:

- Mr SF is a 37 year old man
- married with 2 young children
- he works as an administrator for a logistics company, mainly office-based
- his dad died 6 months ago of a fatal MI; this prompted him to see his GP for a health check – his cholesterol was high
- he was told to reduce his cholesterol by changing his diet, taking more exercise and losing weight; he found dieting difficult; hence 2 weeks ago, he started a Slighter Lite programme of pre-prepared meals
- he had severe foot pain 2 years ago; he was told it was gout, but the follow-up blood test did not show a raised plasma urate so he is confused about the original diagnosis

2. He is seeing the doctor today because:

- he has severe pain in his right foot – he started taking ibuprofen 400 mg thrice daily because he suspected gout, but the foot remains painful; he wants stronger analgesia
- he is confused by the plasma urate test result – does he have gout even if the urate level was normal?
- he feels frustrated as the foot pain has interrupted his exercise programme; he finds dieting difficult as it is and feels angry with this further set-back to his weight loss programme
- if questioned about the Slighter Lite programme, he tells you it is a very low calorie, low carbohydrate diet; he is getting on well with it, having lost 9 kg in 2 weeks
- he is worried about his raised cholesterol because of his dad's fatal MI 6 months ago.
- he expects the doctor to give him advice about gout, to prescribe analgesia, to advise him on when to repeat his blood tests, and to specify which tests are needed and why

Approach to be taken

A. Data gathering, examination and clinical assessment skills

1. *Define the clinical problem: clarify why the patient has presented today*
   The doctor:
   - makes use of the medical records provided; notices the family history, raised cholesterol, history of gout with a normal serum urate from 2 years ago
   - sees that Mr SF limps in and has a facial expression of pain; he responds to this non-verbal cue immediately, with an appropriate opening sentence such as *"You look as if you have a sore foot"*.
   - asks open questions, such as *"How can I help you today?"* to explore the reasons for Mr SF's presentation today
   - asks closed questions, such as *"On a scale of 1–10, how severe is the pain?"* and *"Where exactly is the pain?"* to clarify details of the foot pain
   - works through a diagnostic sieve to exclude other causes of foot pain (such as trauma or Morton's neuroma) and excludes red flags (septic arthritis or rheumatoid arthritis) by asking *"Are you unwell in yourself? Any temperature symptoms or general body aches?"*
   - elicits how the problem is affecting the patient, his family, or his work: *"Were you able to work with this? How are you managing at home?"*
   - discovers Mr SF's ideas: *"I see from your notes you had gout 2 years ago. Do you think this might be gout?"*
   - discovers Mr SF's concerns: *"What are your concerns about what has happened to you?"*
   - discovers Mr SF's expectations: *"By the end of this consultation, what questions would you like to have had answered?"*
   - discovers Mr SF's health beliefs: *"Am I right in thinking that you doubt the diagnosis of gout because the blood test 2 years ago was normal?"*
   - summarises the problem: *"This sounds like gout, but I would like to examine you. Is that OK?"*

2. *Perform an appropriate physical or mental examination*
   The doctor:
   - performs an appropriate physical examination: number of joints affected, erythema, swelling, tenderness and range of motion; if there is diagnostic doubt, takes the patient's temperature, and explains why the examination is being done
   - performs the examination slickly and with sensitivity
   - explains the examination findings in appropriate language, for example, *"One joint is affected, where the big toe meets the instep; it is red, swollen, warm and painful to touch and move; this is typical of gout"*

B. Clinical management skills

3. *Make an appropriate working diagnosis*
   The doctor:
   - integrates information: recognises conditions associated with gout, such as obesity and hypercholesterolaemia
   - on the basis of probability, makes a clinically sound working diagnosis: understands that serum urate measured during the acute attack may be normal; serum urate should be measured 4–6 weeks after the acute attack has resolved

4. *Explain the problem to the patient using appropriate language*
   The doctor:
   - is patient-centred – uses the patient's ideas and beliefs: *"I can understand why the normal blood test made you doubt the diagnosis of gout, but if the test was done in the middle of the attack, it could be misleading; this looks like gout and we are better off doing the test for gout 6 weeks after this episode settles"*
   - paces the explanation appropriately – *"How do you feel about us sorting the pain out now and doing the blood tests later?"*
   - provides information in adequate chunks and checks understanding at each step – *"Did you know that a diet with lots of meat and alcohol can cause gout?"*; after Mr SF responds, the doctor could then say *"Actually, crash dieting with high protein / low carb. diets can also precipitate gout"*
   - addresses the patient's concerns about his difficulty in losing weight – *"Congratulations on losing 9 kg; this shows motivation and hard work, but do you think this type of eating is sustainable? Could you make smaller changes that you could incorporate into your daily routine?"*
   - addresses the patient's expectations – prescribes an NSAID to be used until 48 hours after the acute attack has resolved – and gives the patient the option: does he want a particular tablet he's used successfully in the past?
   - summarises the problem – *"This looks like gout, which we'll treat using an anti-inflammatory tablet. I'll let you think about whether you want to stop the Slighter Lite diet, but I think it's probably precipitated this attack. We'll confirm if it's gout with a blood test in 6 weeks. It may be useful to repeat your cholesterol and fasting glucose tests at the same time."*
   - actively confirms the patient's understanding of the problem – *"We've discussed quite a lot today. So that I know I've explained properly, could you summarise the plan for me?"*

5. *Provide holistic care and use resources effectively*
   The doctor:
   - makes balanced plans which are either doctor or patient-centred as appropriate – negotiates analgesia, and advises on diet and alcohol intake without hectoring or preaching to the patient

- refers appropriately to the Primary Health Care Team (such as the phlebotomist) and other agencies (such as a dietician) if needed
- practises evidence-based medicine and is informed by national or local guidelines, such as: www.cks.library.nhs.uk/gout/view_whole_topic_review

6. *Prescribe appropriately*
The doctor:
- chooses cost-effective medication, such as diclofenac, indometacin or naproxen, with or without paracetamol and codeine
- discusses medication side effects
- checks the patient's understanding of the medication

7. *Specify the conditions and interval for follow-up*
The doctor:
- safety-nets appropriately: *"If you take the tablets regularly and there is no improvement in the pain within 3 days, could you come back to see me?"*

C. Interpersonal skills: know and treat this patient

8. *Achieve rapport*
The doctor:
- listens attentively, picking up the patient's pain, frustration and uncertainty about the diagnosis, and displays empathy to any adverse psychosocial consequences – *"I can see how you thought this diet would be the solution"*
- uses the patient's ideas about the blood test in his explanations
- addresses the patient's specific concerns about weight management and expectations for acute treatment with appropriate NSAIDs / analgesia

9. *Give the patient the opportunity to be involved in significant management decisions*
The doctor:
- shares thoughts and involves the patient in decisions – *"Any ideas about which painkillers work best for you?"*
- negotiates with the patient – *"I think your low carb. diet may be precipitating this. What do you think? Where can you find more information about the side-effects of this diet?"*
- offers choices or various treatment options – *"I can start with a very potent NSAID and step down, or I could start with a potent one and if it doesn't work, you could combine it with paracetamol. Which option would you prefer?"*
- encourages autonomy and opinions – *"Have a think and decide how you want to manage your weight long term"*

Debrief

Discuss how the doctor could, if needed, improve his performance. In particular, assess whether the doctor:

- established good rapport? If so, which behaviour created rapport? Which statements were particularly useful in achieving rapport?
- presented the patient with appropriate treatment options? Did the doctor risk-assess appropriately prior to prescribing? Did the doctor give appropriate lifestyle advice?
- signposted appropriately? For example, prior to examining, did he ask, *"I'd like to examine you now, is that OK?"*
- summarised appropriately? *"This looks like gout, which we'll treat using an anti-inflammatory tablet. I'll let you think about whether you want to stop the Slighter Lite diet, but I think it's probably precipitated this attack. We'll confirm if it's gout with a blood test in 6 weeks. It may be useful to repeat your cholesterol and fasting glucose tests at the same time."*

If the consultation over-ran:

- was the doctor systematic in his history taking? Did he repeat questions? Did he allow the patient to ramble on uninterrupted?
- were the doctor's explanations simple and non-judgemental?

Revising data gathering

What questions could the doctor ask to discover the patient's ideas, concerns, expectations and health beliefs?

- Ideas: *"What do you think has caused this attack of foot pain?"*
- Concerns: *"Was there anything you were particularly worried about?"*
- Expectations: *"Am I right in thinking you'd like some strong painkillers?"*
- Health beliefs: *"It seems to me that you are slightly confused by the normal blood test result you had two years ago. Shall we discuss how gout is diagnosed in more detail?"*

Test your theoretical knowledge

For each of the following statements, answer true (T) or false (F).

1. Advise patients with gout to avoid purine-rich foods, such as bananas, chocolate and tuna.
2. Consider prophylactic medication with colchicine if a person is having two or more attacks of gout in a year.
3. Seek specialist advice if gout occurs during pregnancy.
4. Seek specialist advice if gout occurs in a person less than 25 years of age.
5. Stop allopurinol during an acute attack of gout.

Relevant literature

www.cks.library.nhs.uk/gout/view_whole_topic_review

http://arthritis.about.com/od/gout/a/foodstoeat.htm

Case 8 – Achilles tendinosis

Brief to the doctor

Mr GH is a 33 year old man who consults because of an Achilles tendon problem and would like a referral letter to a private physiotherapist.

Patient summary

Name   GH

Date of birth (Age)   33

Social and family history   Married
                                Estate agent
                                Marathon runner

Past medical history   Nil relevant

Current medication   Ibuprofen 400 mg prn

Tasks for the doctor

In this case, the tasks are to:
- clarify and assess the patient's symptoms
- negotiate an appropriate management plan

Brief to the patient – more about the patient

1. Profile:

- GH is a 33 year old estate agent
- married with 2 children aged 7 and 5 years
- he has run the London marathon for charity for the last 5 years and trains 6 days a week
- 4 months ago he started to notice a gradual onset of pain and stiffness in his left calf on waking and this was eased by a hot shower or by walking; this pain has become more severe and it is now interfering with his running

2. He is seeing the doctor today because:

- having researched the subject on the internet and in running magazines, he would like a letter of referral to a private physiotherapist he has located who specialises in sports injuries. He requires the letter in order to recoup the fees on his private health insurance.

3. Additional information:

- If the doctor asks specifically:
  - the onset of symptoms coincided with changing his running route to include hills, as he wanted to increase the workload and decrease the miles covered so that his training was less time-consuming
  - he has had the same running shoes for 7 months – he has always bought anti-pronation running shoes following an assessment in a specialist running footwear shop
- He believes GPs have no expertise in sports medicine and are not sympathetic to the demands of athletes; consequently:
  - he believes this consultation is a waste of time and he is annoyed that he has to see a doctor just to get a referral letter to someone he is paying to see
  - he is not prepared to take any medication or advice from the doctor
  - he is not prepared to be examined
- He is concerned that he will develop a chronic problem that will end his running days completely.

Approach to be taken

A. Data gathering, examination and clinical assessment skills

1. Define the clinical problem: clarify why the patient has presented today
The doctor:
- reads the patient information provided prior to the consultation
- asks open questions to explore and clarify Mr GH's symptoms and what he has learned about the condition from his research on the internet and in magazines
- empathises with his frustration at the restriction of his running schedule
- asks closed questions to clarify details about possible predisposing factors that might require specific treatment or further referral
- discovers Mr GH's belief that GPs have no expertise in sports injuries and are not sympathetic to athletes when they are injured
- uses internal summaries: *"Can I just recap to make sure I have got things right?"*

2. Performs an appropriate physical or mental examination
- In this case, an examination would normally be performed, but the patient refuses to be examined.
- The need for an examination is explained in appropriate language – *"I would like to examine you in order to ensure that physiotherapy treatment is appropriate before I make a referral."*

B. Clinical management skills

3. Make an appropriate working diagnosis
- The doctor, based on the history, makes a working diagnosis of Achilles tendinopathy.

4. Explain the problem to the patient using appropriate language
The doctor:
- asks *"What do you know about this problem?"*
- asks *"Does my explanation make sense? Is there anything else you would like to know?"*
- explains why private insurers require referral letters

5. Provide holistic care and use resources effectively
- The doctor understands socioeconomic/cultural background: *"It must be very frustrating not being able to run like you used to"*

6. Prescribe appropriately
- The doctor agrees that a physiotherapy referral is appropriate in the first instance and that a physiotherapist with a special interest would be especially beneficial.

7. *Specify the conditions and interval for follow-up*
   - The doctor offers a follow-up appointment if Mr GH does not respond to physiotherapy.

C. Interpersonal skills: know and treat this patient

8. *Achieve rapport*
   The doctor:
   - listens attentively to Mr GH's concerns about his condition
   - explores and clarifies Mr GH's beliefs about GPs' competence in managing sports injuries, but is non-confrontational and non-judgemental
   - understands his request for referral to a specialist physiotherapist
   - shows empathy with Mr GH over his frustration at not being able to train normally and with having to see a doctor for a referral letter

9. *Give the patient the opportunity to be involved in significant management decisions*
   The doctor:
   - actively confirms the patient's understanding of the problem – *"Can I check what you have found out about your problem?"*
   - shares thoughts/involves patient – *"I think you're right to want to see a specialist physio as this problem can be difficult to treat"*

Debrief

Discuss how the doctor could, if needed, improve his performance. In particular, assess how the doctor:

- establishes rapport
- deals with Mr GH's beliefs about GPs' knowledge of sports injuries and sympathy with athletes
- deals with Mr GH's anger at having to consult in order to get a referral letter

Revising data gathering

What questions could the doctor ask to discover the patient's ideas, concerns, expectations and health beliefs?

- Ideas: "*You have done some research for yourself; what have you learned about treatments for your condition?*"
- Concerns: "*Are you worried about the long-term effects of your condition?*"
- Expectations: "*Would you like to ask me about treatments other than physiotherapy?*"
- Health beliefs: "*You don't seem to be very happy about having to see me today, is there a reason for that?*"

Test your theoretical knowledge

For each of the following statements, answer true (T) or false (F).

1. Some antibiotics have been linked with tendinopathies
2. Achilles tendinopathy usually has a good prognosis
3. When examined there is always an area of tenderness and thickening
4. In the acute phase, a 7–15 mm heel raise may relieve pain
5. Histopathologically, in tendinosis, there is neovessel development, collagen fibre disarray and an intense inflammatory response
6. Evidence-based treatments include all of the following: heel-drop (eccentric) exercises, GTN patches, sclerosing injections, and peritendinous corticosteroid injections.

Relevant literature

Alfredson H, Pietila T, Jonsson P, Lorentzon R. (1988) Heavy-load eccentric calf muscle training for the treatment of chronic Achilles tendinosis. *Am J Sports Med,* **26:** 360–366.

Alfredson H, Khan K, Cook J. (2006) An algorithm for managing Achilles tendinopathy: a primary care emphasis on treatment. *Physician Sports Med,* **34**

Case 9 – Heel pain

Brief to the doctor

Mr TP is a 28 year old man who presents with a painful left heel. He says that he saw your colleague, Dr Brown, 3 weeks ago and was told he would be referred to physiotherapy. When he phoned the local physiotherapy unit, he was informed that they hadn't received his referral. He still has heel pain.

Patient summary

Name	TP
Date of birth (Age)	28
Social and Family History	Married, with a baby aged 8 weeks
Past medical history	Insurance medical for mortgage 2 years ago – nil of note
Acute medication	Diclofenac 50 mg thrice daily x 60 tablets

Consultation note by Dr Brown (three weeks ago):
'Actuary with gradual onset (4 weeks) L heel pain, worse medially. Started with morning pain and worse after activity. Now unable to finish rugby game over weekend because of 8/10 pain – walked off field. O/E: tender anterior to heel. Impression: typical plantar fasciitis. Plan: diclofenac x 60T and refer to physiotherapy.' (However, there is no referral letter attached to the consultation.)

Tasks for the doctor

In this case, the tasks are to:
- review what has happened since his previous consultation
- decide whether you need to re-examine
- clarify Mr TP's expectations of this consultation and if appropriate, try to meet them

Brief to the patient – more about the patient

1. Profile:

- Mr TP is a 28 year old actuary who works in the city centre
- he commutes to work by train; this is a busy service and occasionally he has to stand for 20 minutes before he can get a seat.
- married with 1 child, aged 8 weeks – she wakes at night and he has to help bottle-feed; he finds the night walking with baby painful
- Mr TP has never been ill before and is worried about his foot; he assumed he would make a quick recovery once he rested the foot for a couple of weeks

2. He is seeing the doctor today because:

- he called the physiotherapy unit to initiate an appointment and found out they hadn't received a referral letter – he wants to know what happened
- his foot still hurts despite rest and ice for 3 weeks – what should he do?
- he was informed by one of his rugby colleagues that an X-ray may be needed to see if he has a heel spur – should he have an X-ray?

3. Additional information:

- if the doctor does not offer him a suitable explanation or apology for what happened to his referral, he becomes increasingly irritated and overtly unhappy
- if the doctor offers him a private referral, he asks if the practice will pay for it as they inadvertently delayed his treatment
- if the doctor offers him a follow-up appointment in the surgery for a steroid injection, he asks for the risks and benefits and chooses not to have this done
- if the doctor gives him advice that will help him while he waits for his NHS physiotherapy appointment, he leaves feeling 'something has been done' and appears slightly appeased

Approach to be taken

A. Data gathering, examination and clinical assessment skills

1. *Define the clinical problem: clarify why the patient has presented today*
   The doctor:
   - reads the patient information provided prior to the consultation and is alerted by the absence of a referral letter
   - asks open questions to explore what Mr TP expects of today's consultation, thereby eliciting a history of the missing physiotherapy referral and on-going left heel pain
   - acknowledges both issues and empathises with his feelings of anxiety and frustration, for example, *"The absence of a referral letter both at the physiotherapy department and here in your notes does not look too promising, does it? I can see how you could be feeling worried about being let down. I don't know what has happened, but I promise you I will look into it and try to resolve this as best I can. Now, I haven't seen you before so I need to ask you some questions so that I can help you."*
   - asks closed questions to clarify details about the current symptoms and treatments tried
   - excludes red flags such as morning stiffness, back and buttock pain, and tenderness in ligament insertions in the extremities (symptoms of Reiter's disease or ankylosing spondylitis – a small minority of these patients present with plantar fasciitis); this set of questions could be signposted by saying, *"To rule out serious illness I need to ask you a few quick questions. Are your joints stiff in the morning; do you have pain in the…"*
   - explores the impact of the symptoms on his work and home life
   - discovers Mr TP's idea that plantar fasciitis should improve within 3 weeks, especially if the foot is rested and NSAIDs taken
   - discovers Mr TP's concern about having to wait even longer for an NHS physiotherapy appointment
   - discovers Mr TP's expectation of practical help in alleviating the pain and aiding recovery

2. *Performs an appropriate physical or mental examination*
   - In this case, because the history and examination findings of the previous consultation are so typical of plantar fasciitis, an examination is not required.
   - However, if examined, the patient is tender in front of the left heel.
   - The foot may have a high arch or may be flat (pes cavus or planus).
   - When walking, the medial arch (observed from behind) drops, creating a flat foot that rolls in (see www.sportsinjuryclinic.net/cybertherapist/front/foot/plantarfaciitis.htm).
   - Mr TP does not appear to be overweight.

B. Clinical management skills

3. *Make an appropriate working diagnosis*
   - The doctor, based on the typical history, makes a working diagnosis of plantar fasciitis.

4. *Explain the problem to the patient using appropriate language*
   The doctor:
   - having established that Mr TP knows about plantar fasciitis from his previous consultation, addresses his agenda
   - suggests that his idea that plantar fasciitis resolves quickly may be optimistic: studies show that most cases resolve by 6–12 months, but 5% of patients end up undergoing surgery for plantar fascia release when conservative measures fail (www.emedicine.com/EMERG/topic429_4.htm)
   - negotiates a physiotherapy referral; offer to add in a paragraph explaining that the patient had consulted 3 weeks ago and the original referral is missing. Ask Mr TP if he could be available for short notice appointments if other patients cancel and indicate his availability and/or flexibility on the referral document.
   - address his expectation of practical advice: discuss footwear, orthotics, silicone heel pads, steroid injections, self massage by rolling the foot on a golf ball, stretching and strengthening exercises (www.aafp.org/afp/20010201/467.html); advise discontinuation of NSAIDs beyond 10 days
   - provides some information on the pros and cons of steroid injection – potential risks include rupture of the plantar fascia and fat pad atrophy
   - provides information on X-rays: plantar fasciitis produces heel spurs; heel spurs do not produce plantar fasciitis, hence, the spur, if present, should not be surgically removed; an X-ray may not add to the management

5. *Provide holistic care and use resources effectively*
   The doctor:
   - practises evidence-based medicine (www.emedicine.com/EMERG/topic429_4.htm)
   - if Mr TP has a good basic understanding of plantar fasciitis, the doctor should build on this knowledge by discussing exercises (foot biomechanics) and self-help treatments

6. *Prescribe appropriately*
   The doctor:
   - checks the patient's understanding of NSAIDs, efficacy and side effects. The doctor suggests appropriate alternative analgesia.

7. *Specify the conditions and interval for follow-up*
   - The doctor offers a follow-up appointment, either to provide a steroid injection or to discuss any issues arising from the physiotherapy.

C. Interpersonal skills: know and treat this patient

8. *Achieve rapport*
The doctor:
- listens attentively to Mr TP's opening statements and acknowledges his feelings of fear, anxiety and frustration
- deals with his anger at the 'lost' referral without placing undue blame on other members of staff
- displays empathy with regard to the duration of illness and its adverse consequences
- addresses the patient's specific concerns and expectations and encourages self-help

9. *Give the patient the opportunity to be involved in significant management decisions*
- The doctor encourages autonomy and opinions – provides him with treatment options, discusses their risks and benefits and facilitates the patient's choice.

Debrief

Discuss how the doctor could, if needed, improve his performance. In particular, assess whether the doctor:

- was able to able to ask the appropriate 'red flag' questions?
- discussed prognosis? If so, was the language used simple and understandable?
- checked the patient's understanding? How did the doctor do this?
- established rapport and defused the patient's anger? If so, how?

If the consultation over-ran, did the doctor:

- re-take a history of the original presentation instead of focussing on what had happened in the interim?
- perform unnecessary examinations or take too long to examine?
- spend too much time placating the 'angry' patient and too little time addressing his need for on-going treatment?

Revising data gathering

What questions could the doctor ask to discover the patient's ideas, concerns, expectations and health beliefs?

- Ideas: *"How long, do you think, it takes for plantar fasciitis to get better?"*
- Concerns: *"The physiotherapy department has not received your referral. What do you suspect has happened?"*
- Expectations: *"You seem to have a good understanding of plantar fasciitis. What specific issues would you like me to address in today's consultation?"*
- Health beliefs: *"You mentioned getting an X-ray to look for heel spurs. Let's discuss this further"*

Test your theoretical knowledge

For each of the following statements, answer true (T) or false (F).

Regarding plantar fasciitis:

1. The pain is usually caused by collagen deposition at the origin of the plantar fascia at the lateral tubercle of the calcaneus.
2. The worst pain occurs with the first few steps in the morning.
3. Patients often notice pain at the end of activity that lessens or resolves as they rest.
4. Flat feet increases the risk for developing plantar fasciitis while high arches are protective.
5. The pain may be exacerbated by passive dorsiflexion of the toes.
6. The pain may be exacerbated by having the patient stand on the tips of the toes.
7. With age, running shoes retain their shock absorption; getting a new pair of shoes is likely to stretch the arch and increase the pain.
8. Some studies suggest that arch taping and orthotics may be better than NSAIDs or cortisone injection.

Relevant literature

www.aafp.org/afp/20010201/467.html

Case 10 – Acne

Brief to the doctor

Mr GH is a 24 year old man who consults because he has acne affecting his face and back.

Patient summary

Name	GH
Date of birth (Age)	24
Social and family history	Single Labourer
Past medical history	GP consultations: 14 months ago – *"Acne – face and shoulders. Pustules > comedones. For oxytetracycline 250 mg 2 bd 3/12"* 11 months ago – *"Acne review. No improvement after 3/12 oxytet, add benzoyl peroxide gel. Warned re irritation and bleaching."*
Current medication	None No recorded allergies
Investigations	None

Tasks for the doctor

In this case, the tasks are to:
- review previous medication and try to identify why he has not responded
- identify Mr GH's concerns about his acne and offer support
- prescribe appropriately

Brief to the patient – more about the patient

1. Profile:

- Mr GH is a 24 year old single man
- he works as a labourer on a building site

2. He is seeing the doctor today because:

- he has had acne (spots and blackheads) on his face and back for just over a year and is concerned about the cosmetic appearance
- he saw a GP last year and was given a 3 month course of oxytetracycline without any real benefit; benzoyl peroxide was then added, but again this did not help; he did not bother going back
- he is training to take part in a body building competition – he feels he will not score well in the competition if he is 'spotty'

3. Additional information:

- He was not troubled by acne as a teenager; his voice broke age 11 and he started shaving at 14, by which age he was 6' 1" tall.
- If the doctor asks specifically:
  - he does not come into contact with any chemicals at work
  - for the last 18 months he has been using protein supplements which he buys at the gym
  - most of the other body builders at the gym use steroid tablets and injections
  - he follows a high protein high carbohydrate diet
  - his girlfriend recently split up with him after 4 years together because she was fed up with him always being at the gym and said that he had been become moody and snappy
  - he is not sleeping well; he has no depressive symptoms
- He believes he can train and do well 'naturally'; he refuses to use steroids because he has heard they have long-term effects that are irreversible.
- His trainer has pressured him on several occasions to use steroids. Taking the protein supplements was a compromise that Mr GH complied with to get his trainer 'off his back'.
- He is not aware that some supplements have been reported to contain traces of androgenic-anabolic steroids.
- If the doctor performs an examination:

System	Findings
General	Very well built fit young man No jaundice. No gynaecomastia. Normal body hair
Skin	Comedones and pustules on face, shoulders and back. No scarring or cysts.
Cardiovascular	BP 134/88 (use large cuff)
Abdomen	No enlarged liver No evidence of testicular atrophy

Approach to be taken

A. Data gathering, examination and clinical assessment skills

1. *Define the clinical problem: clarify why the patient has presented today*
   The doctor:
   - reads the patient information provided prior to the consultation
   - asks open questions to explore:
     - whether Mr GH had acne in the past and how it was treated
     - why he is concerned about his acne at this time
     - whether the acne is having any psychosocial effects on him– "*How is this affecting you?*"
     - whether Mr GH has considered that the protein supplements might contain traces of androgenic-anabolic steroids and that this might be the cause of his acne – "*Some sports supplements have been found to contain traces of anabolic steroids and other substances – have you ever wondered about this?*"
   - asks closed questions to:
     - exclude other causes of rashes – "*As a builder, do you come into contact with any irritant chemicals that might cause this?*"
     - be sure that he is not knowingly using androgenic-anabolic steroids or other agents – "*I am sorry, but I have to ask this question because it will affect how we treat your problem. Are you taking any supplements or other substances to enhance your performance or physique?*"
     - assess if he has experienced other possible unwanted effects of androgenic-anabolic steroids – psychological
   - empathises with Mr GH about:
     - the cosmetic effects and having acne occur for the first time at his age rather than in his teens: "*It must be a bit of a shock starting to get acne as an adult rather than as a teenager. How are you coping with that?*"
     - his feelings about androgenic-anabolic steroid use: "*You have heard that anabolic steroids have some serious side-effects, would you like to discuss this?*"

2. *Performs an appropriate physical or mental examination*
   - In this case, a targeted examination is required. A minimally acceptable examination would be, with the patient's shirt removed:
     - examination of the acne to confirm the diagnosis and assess severity
     - a quick visual check to exclude gynaecomastia, loss of body hair, and liver disease stigmata
   - If time permits, a BP check could be done, although this could be deferred to a follow up appointment, given that there are no other signs of anabolic steroid use.
   - The need for an examination should be explained in appropriate language.

B. Clinical management skills

3. *Make an appropriate working diagnosis*
   - The doctor integrates information and makes a working diagnosis of acne probably secondary to androgenic-anabolic steroid use.
   - This is a clinically sound hypothesis with an appropriate use of probability.

4. *Explain the problem to the patient using appropriate language*
   The doctor:
   - having established Mr GH's feelings about drugs, sensitively explains that some protein supplements have been reported to contain androgenic-anabolic steroids – *"If I were to say to you that some supplements have been reported to contain anabolic steroids, how would you feel?"*
   - explains that acne is a reported unwanted effect of androgenic-anabolic steroids
   - provides information on androgenic-anabolic steroids to include unwanted effects
   - advises Mr GH that the unwanted effects are largely reversible if androgenic-anabolic steroid use is stopped
   - uses chunking and checking of information to evaluate Gary's understanding: *"I have given you a lot of unexpected information, before I examine you, can I just check that I have explained things clearly?"*

5. *Provide holistic care and use resources effectively*
   The doctor:
   - builds on Mr GH's health beliefs to identify management options – *"You've told me that you are against drugs, would you be happy to stop using the supplements and see if the problem goes away?"*
   - understands socioeconomic/cultural background – *"Are you concerned that stopping the supplements might affect your chances in the competition?"*
   - discusses with Mr GH whether to perform blood tests to look for biochemical effects of androgenic-anabolic steroids – *"It is possible that you may have been taking a supplement that contains steroids and that this is the cause of your acne. We have talked about some of the side effects of these. Would you like to have a blood test to check whether there are any signs of other side effects?"*

6. *Prescribe appropriately*
   - The doctor agrees an appropriate management plan with the patient to include:
     - that Mr GH should stop taking the protein supplements and be reviewed in a month to see if his acne had improved
     - having blood tests – FBC, U&Es, LFTs, fasting glucose and fasting lipids

7. *Specify the conditions and interval for follow-up*
   - The doctor arranged a follow-up appointment to monitor progress of the acne and review the blood test results.

C. Interpersonal skills: know and treat this patient

8. *Achieve rapport*
   The doctor:
   - listens attentively
   - follows up verbal and non-verbal cues – *"You mentioned body-building, I know that some body builders use special supplements to improve their performance..."*
   - sensitively explores and clarifies Mr GH's supplement use and his feelings about androgenic-anabolic steroids
   - places the problem in a psychosocial context – how it affects patient/ relationships: *"You mentioned that your girlfriend said you were moody and snappy, was this just with her?"*
   - is non-judgemental about Mr GH's use of protein supplements
   - empathises with Mr GH about getting acne in adult life

9. *Give the patient the opportunity to be involved in significant management decisions*
   The doctor:
   - actively confirms patient's understanding of the problem – *"Is there anything else you would like to ask?"*
   - shares thoughts with the patient that the protein supplements may be causing the acne
   - encourages autonomy by building on Mr GH's ideas and concerns about taking anabolic steroids to agree a management plan

Debrief

Discuss how the doctor could, if needed, improve his performance. In particular, assess how the doctor:
- established rapport and identified Mr GH's beliefs about androgenic-anabolic steroid use
- raised the possibility of the supplements containing androgenic-anabolic steroids and that this might be the cause of his acne

Revising data gathering

What questions could the doctor ask to discover the patient's ideas, concerns, expectations and health beliefs?
- Ideas: "*I understand that you are surprised that you have started getting acne at your age, do you have any ideas why this has happened now?*"
- Concerns: "*Are you concerned that you might have other side effects of anabolic steroids?*"
- Expectations: "*Would you like to have some blood tests to see if there are any signs of other steroid side effects?*"
- Health beliefs: "*You said that you are worried about the long-term effects of androgenic-anabolic steroids, would you like to discuss this?*"

Test your theoretical knowledge

For each of the following statements, answer true (T) or false (F).
1. The requirements for protein and calories appear to increase when training with the aid of anabolic-androgenic steroids
2. Anabolic-androgenic steroids remain detectable for several weeks whether taken orally or by injection
3. Drugs on the World Anti-Doping Agency 'banned list' include all beta 2 agonists, tamoxifen, and thiazide diuretics
4. Anabolic-androgenic steroids may induce hyperinsulinism
5. Regimens for using anabolic-androgenic steroids include stacking, pyramids, and tapering
6. Before more effective drugs were available, anabolic-androgenic steroids had been used to treat depression and other mental health disorders

Relevant literature

Bahrke MS, Yesalis CE. (2002) *Performance-Enhancing Substances in Sport and Exercise.* Human Kinetics, Champaign Illinois.

World Anti-Doping Agency (WADA) website: www.wada-ama.org

WADA Athlete guide:
www.wada-ama.ork/rtecontent/document/WADA_Athlete-Guide_ENG.pdf

Case 11 – Post-partum problems

Brief to the doctor

Mrs PH is a 32 year old woman who is added to the end of your clinic as a telephone consultation. You call her back on the number supplied. Mrs PH saw the practice nurse 4 days ago for blood tests.

Patient summary

Name	PH
Date of birth (Age)	34
Social and Family History	Married with two children Her son was born 10 days ago
Past medical history	Heartburn during pregnancy
Current medication	Gaviscon as required

Consultation note by practice nurse (four days ago):
'Discharged from labour ward but advised to have FBC taken as loss of 850 ml blood. Is feeling light-headed but not SOB. Blood taken from L cubital fossa using aseptic technique. Patient advised to call surgery for results in 3–5 days.'

Blood tests	Tests were done four days ago
Hb	10.5 g/dl (12–15)
MCV	97 (83–105)
White cell count	6.67 (4–11)
Differential count	no abnormalities
Platelet count	285 (150–400)

Tasks for the doctor

In this case, the tasks are to:
- clarify, with attention to auditory cues, Mrs PH's reason(s) for calling
- take a detailed history
- actively confirm that the patient understands the treatment plan

Brief to the patient – more about the patient

1. Profile:

- Mrs PH is a 34 year old woman who is currently on maternity leave; her baby boy was born 10 days ago
- she is married and has an older daughter, aged 6
- Mrs PH wants the results of her blood tests; she was also advised by the health visitor to tell you about the 'clot' she has passed

2. She is calling the doctor today because:

- she would like to know the results of her recent blood tests and whether treatment is needed
- the health visitor advised her to tell the GP about the clot she passed: two days ago, she passed one small clot vaginally – it was the size of a 50 pence coin; the clot did not seem to contain any tissue and there have not been other clots or smelly discharge or abdominal pain
- when asked about the birth, she tells you that her waters broke at 2 pm, her labour progressed quickly, her baby was born by NVD at 10 pm, but she was then taken to theatre for a manual removal of placenta, hence the 850 ml loss of blood; she cannot remember if the she was given antibiotics intravenously at the time of the procedure and she was not given antibiotic tablets after the manual removal
- she feels well in herself and has not had fever or rigors
- her main concern is that treatments may interfere with her breastfeeding; she has had a few problems with breastfeeding, which is why she is seeing the health visitor for advice – she wants to breastfeed and would prefer to avoid formula milk if at all possible; she is wary of antibiotics, particularly if antibiotics pass into breast milk and give the baby diarrhoea, resulting in further weight loss
- she expects advice: what should she do about her blood results and her bleeding?

3. Additional information:

- if the doctor discusses an iron-rich diet, she says that she eats meat, bran, baked beans, etc. and has no problem avoiding tea and coffee with meals
- if the doctor suggests iron tablets, she says she has not had problems with iron tablets in the past – she expects the doctor to make arrangements for the prescription
- if you suggest a wait and see policy, she expects to be told when to seek your advice again
- if you suggest that she comes in to see a GP, she wants to know if she needs to attend today as arranging childcare for her 6 year old may be difficult

Approach to be taken

A. Data gathering, examination and clinical assessment skills

1. *Define the clinical problem: clarify why the patient has telephoned today*
   The doctor:
   - reads the patient information provided prior to the consultation and notes that Mrs HP lost 850 ml of blood during birth and now has an Hb of 10.6 g/dl
   - telephones Mrs HP on the number provided; he introduces himself and establishes the identity of the patient – if someone else answers, he asks to speak to the patient because a first-hand history is usually more reliable
   - clarifies the nature of the problem and understands exactly what the patient is requesting today; one approach is *"I see from your notes you recently gave birth. Congratulations! I also see that you had some blood tests done a few days ago. What can I do for you today?"*
   - asks open questions to explore the two issues raised by the patient, such as *"How are you feeling now?"* or *"Tell me more about the clots"*
   - asks closed questions to clarify details about the post-partum bleeding: fever, rigors, feeling unwell, racing pulse, risk factors for endometritis, such as a manual removal of placenta; by asking about current infection, the doctor systematically excludes red flags signalling the need for review or referral
   - empathises with her difficulties in breastfeeding and elicits her concerns regarding treatments that may interfere with breastfeeding
   - elicits her expectations for advice regarding her two issues, namely anaemia and post-partum bleeding

2. *Performs an appropriate physical or mental examination*
   - In this case, an examination is not required. The difficulty with telephone triage is the ability to make management decisions in the absence of visual cues.

B. Clinical management skills

3. *Make an appropriate working diagnosis*
   - The doctor, based on the history, makes a working diagnosis of (1) anaemia due to blood loss at delivery, and (2) the possibility of secondary post-partum haemorrhage (PPH) due to endometrial infection.

4. *Explain the problem to the patient using appropriate language*
   The doctor:
   - addresses Mrs PH's agenda: what does Mrs PH know about dietary treatments for anaemia / iron tablets / fluids that reduce iron absorption? The doctor may explain why he is concerned about the PV bleeding – that it could be a warning sign of 'hidden infection in the womb'

- gives the information about PPH in digestable chunks: a severe case of PPH would have more bleeding or purulent lochia, the patient would feel unwell (like flu), have a racing pulse, feel flushed and feverish, with sweating that wets the clothes; the patient's understanding is checked at each step
- addresses Mrs PH's concerns: an iron-rich diet, with or without iron tablets, is unlikely to interfere with breastfeeding; further assessment of the vaginal bleed may be needed in the form of a pelvic examination – she may not want her 6 year old daughter present during this examination (or the curtains could be drawn around the bed for privacy) – the assessment could take place within the next few days, at her convenience; however, if symptoms of severe infection develop, she needs to see a doctor urgently
- 'prescribes' an iron-rich diet and negotiates prescription of iron tablets according to Mrs PH's preferences

5. *Provide holistic care and use resources effectively*
The doctor:
- manages both problems (anaemia and PV bleeding) in accordance with national or local guidelines
- checks that there is agreement and understanding with what is proposed
- does not waste time addressing the breastfeeding issue if Mrs CC is happy with the advice she has received from the health visitor – the time is better spent addressing her concerns about anaemia and PV bleeding

6. *Prescribe appropriately*
The doctor:
- is aware of national and local guidelines – www.nice.org.uk/nicemedia/pdf/CG037fullguideline.pdf (pages 113–125) and www.bsg.org.uk/pdf_word_docs/iron_def.pdf
- if prescribing, discusses how iron tablets are taken and the commonly experienced side effects

7. *Specify the conditions and interval for follow-up*
The doctor:
- arranges the follow-up appointment for the pelvic examination
- outlines the red flag symptoms; if these symptoms develop, Mrs PH should seek urgent care (i.e safety-nets)
- summarises, for example, with *"Just to recap, we've agreed that you will eat more red meat and cornflakes and avoid tea and coffee with meals. Your husband will collect the prescription for iron tablets and you will take one tablet daily with orange juice. You will keep an eye on your vaginal bleeding. If it is settling you will see me for an examination at your convenience in the next few days. If you develop a temperature, more bleeding, or start to feel unwell, you will ring back and I will see you as an emergency appointment. Are you happy with these arrangements?"*

C. Interpersonal skills: know and treat this patient

8. *Achieve rapport*
   The doctor:
   - listens attentively to Mrs PH's request for advice, does not interrupt unnecessarily, and maintains the flow of conversation
   - questions in a systematic manner, taking care to deal with one issue at a time
   - is sensitive in his queries and ensures that the conversation does not sound like an interrogation
   - understands the patient's request for advice and refrains from making comments such as *"I don't know why the health visitor didn't sort this out herself!"*
   - displays empathy to her predicament – *"I can understand why you'd prefer to avoid any tablets that interfere with the breastfeeding routine you've worked so hard to establish. Let me reassure you that iron tablets will not affect the feeding."*
   - is alert to the possibility of PPH in someone who has had a manual removal of the placenta; however, he does not alarm the patient unduly

9. *Give the patient the opportunity to be involved in significant management decisions*
   - The doctor encourages autonomy and opinions – provides the patient with information on diet and iron tablets and allows her to choose her own treatment; provides sufficient information on why a pelvic examination may be needed and Mrs PH is able to make an appointment that fits in with her childcare

Debrief

Discuss how the doctor could, if needed, improve his performance. In particular, assess whether the doctor:
- established rapport on the telephone? If so, how?
- established the patient's reasons for calling? If so, how?
- dealt with Mrs PH's specific concerns in a systematic manner? If so, how?
- discussed the red flags for PPH in a non-alarmist manner?
- summarised and checked understanding?

If the consultation over-ran, did the doctor:
- interrupt unnecessarily?
- get side-tracked by other issues, such as breastfeeding, that Mrs PH was happy to leave to the health visitor?
- repeat some explanations and reassurances?

Revising data gathering

What questions could the doctor ask to discover the patient's ideas, concerns, expectations and health beliefs?
- Ideas: *"Do you have any ideas on how anaemia (low blood counts) is treated?"*
- Concerns: *"Regarding the clot, did you have any worries about what might be happening?"*
- Expectations: *"It seems to me that you want a treatment that does not interfere with your breastfeeding. Do I understand you correctly?"*
- Health beliefs: *"You sound as if you suspect that something is not quite right if you pass a clot a week after delivering. Let's talk about this for a moment."*

Test your theoretical knowledge

For each of the following statements, answer true (T) or false (F).
1. The WHO classifies anaemia in non-pregnant women, over 15 years, as an Hb < 12 g/dl.
2. The WHO classifies anaemia in pregnant women, as an Hb < 10 g/dl.
3. If iron deficiency anaemia co-exists with a B12 or folate deficiency, the red cell distribution width (RDW) is decreased.
4. Continue oral iron therapy (ferrous sulphate 200 mg twice daily) for three months after the iron deficiency has been corrected to replenish stores.
5. Teenage girls and women under 50 years should have 14.8 mg of iron a day.
6. A 125 g can of sardines in tomato sauce contains less iron than two slices of lean roast beef.
7. A 30 g bowl of branflakes and a 30 g bowl cornflakes contain equivalent amounts of iron.

Relevant literature

www.weightlossresources.co.uk/diet/healthy_diet/iron_rich_food.htm

www.bsg.org.uk/pdf_word_docs/iron_def.pdf

Case 12 – Relative with bowel cancer

Brief to the doctor

Mr KL is a 20 year old man who presents in a routine surgery. He has registered as a temporary resident as he is in his first year at university. He has come home because his father has recently had surgery for bowel cancer at the age of 44 years. He has asked to talk about genetic screening for bowel cancer with a doctor. Mr KL saw one of your partners last year, just before he left to go to university, when he had noticed some blood on the toilet paper for a few days, but he was told not to worry.

Patient summary

Name	KL
Date of birth (Age)	20
Social and family history	Student Father diagnosed with cancer of the bowel 2 months ago
Past medical history	GP consultation: 1 year ago – *"c/o fresh blood on toilet paper when he wipes – 4 days, none in pan. Stool normal but has been straining a bit. Well in self. No pain. Prob pile. Reassured, told to return if continues."*
Current medication	None
Investigations	None

Tasks for the doctor

In this case, the tasks are to:
- confirm details of his father's diagnosis and any advice given for relatives by the hospital consultant, while respecting KL's father's right to confidentiality; as a result discuss whether Mr KL should be referred for genetic advice and screening
- explore Mr KL's concerns about his rectal bleeding last year
- discuss symptoms and factors linked with bowel cancer, including genetics; discuss any lifestyle changes Mr KL may like to make

Brief to the patient – more about the patient

1. Profile:

- Mr KL is a 20 year old Sports Science student
- he lives in a hall of residence but tends not to eat there as he often goes to the gym in the evenings and so has takeaways or Pot Noodles in the evenings
- he saw one of the GPs in this practice a year ago because he had had some rectal bleeding and was told he probably had a pile and need not worry. He has had a couple of episodes of fresh blood on the paper since then. His health is excellent – he feels well and has not lost weight.
- his father had rectal bleeding 6 months ago and saw the same partner KL saw last year and the father was also told he probably had piles and not to worry – he then saw another partner and was referred to the hospital 2 months ago. Mr KL's father has told him that he had a 'Stage 2' tumour. His father has had a right hemicolectomy and is going to have chemotherapy.
- Mr KL is angry that his father was not referred earlier by your partner and concerned that he had the same symptoms and was also 'fobbed off' without an examination
- Mr KL believes that lifestyle has a major effect on health and is very open to health promotion advice – he feels guilty that he has neglected his own diet
- he has not looked up bowel cancer on the internet yet as he has not had time, but intends to do so

2. He is seeing the doctor today because:

- he wants information on the genetics of bowel cancer and advice on whether he should have screening; he would like to discuss what screening tests are possible and their accuracy
- he would like to be reassured about his own rectal bleeding and would like to be told exactly what the cause is – he feels he should be examined and referred to a specialist
- he wants advice on what preventive measures he can take

3. Addditional information:

- If the doctor examines him:

System	Findings
General	Well. No evidence of weight loss No pallor
Abdomen	Soft. No tenderness No masses or organomegaly
Rectal examination	Perianal skin – NAD. No external piles/skin tags Empty rectum. No masses felt. No blood on glove

Approach to be taken

A. Data gathering, examination and clinical assessment skills

1. *Define the clinical problem: clarify why the patient has presented today*
   The doctor:
   - reads the patient information provided prior to the consultation
   - asks open questions to clarify details of:
     - Mr KL's father's condition – *"I haven't got your father's records, tell me about him."*
     - Mr KL's concerns for himself – *"You seem concerned that you have the same symptoms as your father?"*
     - Mr KL's request for information on genetic screening – *"What do you know about screening for bowel cancer?"*
     - Mr KL's knowledge about causes of the condition
   - asks closed questions to clarify:
     - details of Mr KL's own symptoms to exclude red flag symptoms signalling the need for review or referral
     - what advice, if any, the hospital has given about screening the rest of the family
   - uses internal summaries – *"Can I just check I've got things right..."*

2. *Performs an appropriate physical or mental examination*
   - In this case, an examination is required to address the patient's concerns.
   - The examination should be explained in appropriate language – *"I need to examine your abdomen and then do an internal examination with a finger."*
   - A targeted examination should be performed – abdomen and RE.

B. Clinical management skills

3. *Make an appropriate working diagnosis*
   - The doctor, based on the history and examination, makes a working diagnosis of haemorrhoidal bleeding.
   - This is a clinically sound hypothesis and makes an appropriate use of probability.

4. *Explain the problem to the patient using appropriate language*
   The doctor:
   - explains the likely cause of Mr KL's symptoms
   - addresses Mr KL's agenda:
     - that he should be referred to ensure he does not have cancer
     - discusses factors associated with bowel cancer pertinent to him including diet and genetics: *"What do you know about causes of bowel cancer?"*
     - discusses screening for bowel cancer: *"Do you know much about screening for bowel cancer?"*

- addreses Mr KL's concerns about the management of his father in a non-judgemental way and respecting his father's confidentiality

5. **Provide holistic care and use resources effectively**
The doctor:
- practises evidence-based medicine using national guidelines – NICE (2005) *Referral guidelines for suspected cancer* (CG27 – www.nice.org.uk/Guidance/CG27)
- uses Mr KL's health beliefs to reinforce advice about preventive measures he could take – "*You seem to be keen on preventing cancers, would you like to discuss things you might be able to do to decrease your risks?*"
- respects his father's right to confidentiality – "*I am afraid I can't discuss details of your father's case without his permission. Can I suggest you discuss your concerns with your family to see if they share your feelings?*"
- advises Mr KL about the complaints procedure – "*Would you like me to give you details of how to make a complaint, if you and your family decide to do so?*"

6. **Prescribe appropriately**
The doctor:
- chooses to advise Mr KL about diet rather than provide local treatments (haemorrhoid creams) for the management of his symptoms
- writes to Mr KL's father's consultant to ask if Mr KL should also be referred for screening as his father had developed bowel cancer before the age of 45, with a copy to Mr KL's GP at university for information

7. **Specify the conditions and interval for follow-up**
The doctor:
- offers a follow-up appointment to discuss any issues arising from Mr KL's own symptoms, lifestyle change and his father's condition
- checks understanding: "*Just to check that I have explained things clearly, can you tell me what we have agreed to do today?*"

C. Interpersonal skills: know and treat this patient

8. **Achieve rapport**
The doctor:
- listens attentively to Mr KL's concerns about:
  - his father's condition and perceived delayed referral
  - his own symptoms and his risk of developing bowel cancer in the future
- explores and clarifies Mr KL's health beliefs and concerns – that lifestyle contributes to maintaining health
- understands his request for information on screening and genetic counselling
- is non-judgemental about the patient's ideas on his father's management, but expresses sympathy with Mr KL's feelings and upset

9. *Give the patient the opportunity to be involved in significant management decisions*
The doctor:
- actively confirms the patient's understanding of the problem: *"Does my explanation of the likely cause of your symptoms sound reasonable to you?"*
- balances plans – doctor/patient centred as appropriate – *"I don't think I need to refer you about your bleeding at the moment, but agree it would be sensible to check with the hospital whether your father had one of the sorts of cancer that might have a genetic component, in which case you will need to be referred"*

Debrief

Discuss how the doctor could, if needed, improve his performance. In particular, assess how the doctor:

- obtained information about Mr KL's father's cancer to enable him to answer Mr KL's questions. Did he get all the necessary information from Mr KL or could he have consulted the father's medical records? What are the issues relating to discussing his father's records with Mr KL?
- dealt with Mr KL's rectal bleeding symptoms. Was an examination appropriate or necessary? Should a chaperone be offered?
- dealt with Mr KL's anger over his partner's advice to both Mr KL and his father
- gained Mr KL's trust

Revising data gathering

What questions could the doctor ask to discover the patient's ideas, concerns, expectations and health beliefs?

- Ideas: "*You seem to be angry about the advice the other doctor gave you and your father; would you like to discuss that?*"
- Concerns: "*Are you worried that you might develop bowel cancer at some time in the future?*"
- Expectations: "*You said you were unhappy that my partner didn't examine you last year; would you prefer to be examined today?*" and "*I understand your anxiety about your own symptoms and why you would like an exact diagnosis, how were you hoping I would help with those today?*"
- Health beliefs: "*Being fit and healthy is important to you; would you like to discuss things you can do that might decrease your chances of developing bowel cancer?*"

Once the doctor has gathered sufficient information, how could he summarise the problem for the patient?

- "*We have discussed a lot of things today, can I just summarise them to make sure I have covered all the things you wanted and that we have agreed on what to do about them all?*"
- "*Are you happy with what we have covered or do you have any questions or concerns?*"

Test your theoretical knowledge

For each of the following statements, answer true (T) or false (F).

1. Bowel cancer is the second commonest cause of cancer-related deaths in Western countries
2. Dietary factors play a minimal role in developing bowel cancer
3. Trials have shown that aspirin 300 mg daily reduces the risk of bowel cancer by 20%

4. The commonest inherited form of bowel cancer is non-polyposis colon cancer (HNPCC or Lynch Syndrome)
5. Faecal occult blood (FOB) screening has a sensitivity of 90% for bowel cancers
6. Anyone over 55 with rectal bleeding, or anyone with a combination of rectal bleeding and altered bowel habit, should be seen at a hospital within 2 weeks of referral by their GP

Relevant literature

Jones R, Latinovic R, Charlton J, Gulliford MC. (2007) Alarm symptoms in early diagnosis of cancer in primary care: cohort study using General Practice Research Database. *BMJ*, **334:** 1040–1044.

Departement of Health (2000) *Referral guidelines for suspected cancer.*

NICE (2005) *Referral guidelines for suspected cancer,* CG27: www.nice.org.uk/Guidance/CG27

Case 13 – Food poisoning

Brief to the doctor

Mr EJ is a 32 year old man who consulted your colleague, Dr Brown 5 days ago. The microbiology laboratory telephoned the practice nurse this morning to relay the results of Mr EJ's stool sample: campylobacter was isolated. The nurse added Mr EJ to your appointment list for you to telephone him with the results.

Patient summary

Name	EJ
Date of birth (Age)	32
Social and Family History	Unmarried; works as an airline steward
Past medical history	Low back pain 6 months ago Poor sleep pattern 2 years ago
Medication	None

Dr Brown's consultation (5 days ago)
'Diarrhoea symptoms: frequent, loose motions. Fresh blood from piles and no mucus. Passing watery stool every 1–2 hours. Crampy, abdominal pain – using NSAIDs and paracetamol. Recent travel to Jordan and Germany; stayed in hotels. Ate egg sandwich at Frankfurt airport. Had salmonella age 17. O/E: hydrated, slightly dry lips. Generalised abdominal tenderness. No guarding. T 37.3°C. Plan: get stool samples x 2. Use immodium only if diarrhoea is interrupting sleep. Not due back at work for a few days.'

Tasks for the doctor

In this case, the tasks are to:
- contact Mr EJ with his results
- review his symptoms
- provide appropriate occupational advice

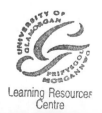

Learning Resources
Centre

Brief to the patient – more about the patient

1. Profile:

- Mr EJ is a 32 year old man who works as a steward for a budget airline
- he is unmarried and lives alone; he has had several relationships with partners of the same sex. His last HIV test at the GUM clinic 3 months ago, after the break-up of his most recent relationship, was negative. He has used condoms since.
- Mr EJ feels ill and is worried about the abdominal cramp he is experiencing with this bout of food poisoning.

2. When the surgery contacts him, he updates them on his illness:

- the diarrhoea has improved but he does not feel completely well
- he passes two to three loose, not watery, stools daily and is now able to sleep through the night; he did not use any tablets to reduce stool frequency – he drank fluids to rehydrate and now tolerates bland food. He does not have nausea or vomiting.
- he still experiences generalised stomach cramp, unrelated to meals, but the cramp is not as severe (3/10) nor does it last as long (10 minutes) compared to 5 days ago
- he has been recuperating at home. However, he is due to fly to Spain on the early flight tomorrow and thinks he feels well enough to undertake the short-haul. He works several flights for the next 3 days after which he meets with friends in Spain where a party is planned.
- he is shocked to hear about the positive campylobacter result; he expected the cultures to be negative, and he wants to know if further treatment is needed
- he expects to return to work tomorrow – is this OK? As a steward, one of his duties is to sell packaged food and beverages on flights.
- does he need to inform work about his results?
- with regard to the party, is he OK to drink alcohol?
- Mr EJ is a chatty man and one of the difficulties in this case is to remain focussed on the relevant medical issues

3. Additional information:

- if the doctor does not prescribe antibiotics, he wants to know if there could be complications later on?
- should he give a stool sample at a later date to check for eradication?
- if the doctor prescribes antibiotics, he wants to know if he can return to work within 24 hours – presumably he won't be infectious then?
- this is his 2nd bowel infection – is there something predisposing him to bowel infections? Is there anything he can do to prevent getting infections?

Approach to be taken

A. Data gathering, examination and clinical assessment skills

1. *Define the clinical problem: inform the patient of the results and clarify the issues a positive result has for him*
   The doctor:
   - reads the patient notes provided prior to the telephone consultation and thinks about what information he needs to obtain from Mr EJ
   - telephones Mr EJ on the number provided and introduces himself; he establishes the identity of the caller / patient and speaks to the patient directly
   - signposts or structures the consultations, for example, says *"Mr EJ, I have the results of your stool sample. Before we discuss these, I'd like to ask you some questions."*
   - asks open questions to explore how Mr EJ is feeling at the moment and, if there has been an improvement, what has improved and what helped him to feel better
   - asks closed questions to clarify details about fever, pain, diarrhoea (frequency, consistency, presence of blood or mucus) since he was last seen
   - asks about red flag symptoms (which may signal the need for antibiotics), namely feeling very unwell, having a high temperature, passing more than eight stools per day, being ill for longer than 1 week or being immunocompromised
   - empathises with the pain and disruption the diarrhoea has caused to Mr EJ's usual routine; clarifies the impact the illness has had on his family and work. The doctor is alert to the fact that Mr EJ is a food handler.
   - discovers Mr EJ's idea that his illness is a mild, self-limiting case of food poisoning, his expectation of returning to work as an airline steward tomorrow, and his concern about whether work should be informed about a positive campylobacter result

2. *Performs an appropriate physical or mental examination*
   - In this case, an examination is not required.

B. Clinical management skills

3. *Make an appropriate working diagnosis*
   - The doctor, based on the history, makes a working diagnosis of improving campylobacter diarrhoea. In the absence of red flag symptoms, antibiotics are not indicated. However, this needs to be balanced against his status as a food handler who, if not given antibiotics, may continue to shed organisms in the stool for up to 4 weeks. Infection usually occurs via infected food or

145

water; person-to-person transmission via the faeco-oral route is rare. In addition, Mr EJ handles packaged food so the risk of transmission is further reduced.

4. *Explain the problem to the patient using appropriate language*
The doctor:
- having established that Mr EJ is improving, informs him of his microbiology results
- provides him with information about the natural history of campylobacter gastroenteritis and possible treatments: rehydration (200 ml after each loose stool), antibiotics in severe cases (erythromycin or ciprofloxin), avoid antimotility drugs, and probiotics may help to reduce the duration of diarrhoea by 1 day
- provides some occupational advice: all workers, including food handlers, are advised to return to work 48 hours after the last episode of diarrhoea
- addresses Mr EJ's specific questions about possible complications (15% develop irritable bowel syndrome post-infection)

5. *Provide holistic care and use resources effectively*
The doctor:
- practises evidence-based medicine that is informed by national or local guidelines
- informs Mr EJ about camplylobacter being a notifiable disease (search for "notifiable diseases" on www.hpa.org.uk)
- if Mr EJ does not raise the issue of a sick note, the doctor (time permitting) may wish to inform him that notes are issued for sickness absences lasting more than 6 days
- some companies offer flexible working patterns and if the patient is unable to attend work (e.g. with diarrhoea), then some work, especially if computer or internet based, can be done from home; patients are encouraged to liaise directly with their occupational health or human resources departments

6. *Prescribe appropriately*
- The doctor is aware of national and local guidelines when making a decision on prescribing (http://cks.library.nhs.uk/mobiledevices/ckscontent.aspx?rawurl=gastroenteritis)

7. *Specify the conditions and interval for follow-up*
The doctor:
- discusses the 'red flag' symptoms and advises the patient to consult if these develop
- if sick certification advice is provided, the advice is in line with national guidance (www.hpa.org.uk/cdph/issues/CDPHvol7/No4/guidelines2_4_04.pdf – see page 368)

C. Interpersonal skills: know and treat this patient

8. *Achieve rapport*
   The doctor:
   - listens attentively to Mr EJ's account of his current symptoms and displays empathy to its adverse impact on his life
   - understands his request for information on the natural history and possible treatments of campylobacter as the patient knows very little about this infection
   - uses his ideas about self-limiting illness in explanations
   - addresses his specific concerns about what to tell work and his expectations of when to resume air stewarding duties

9. *Give the patient the opportunity to be involved in significant management decisions*
   The doctor:
   - discusses the pros and cons of antibiotic and probiotic treatments and negotiates with the patient
   - encourages patient autonomy by providing him with enough information so that he feels able to discuss work issues with his company

Debrief

Discuss how the doctor could, if needed, improve his performance. In particular, assess whether the doctor:

- asked questions in a systematic and structured manner? If so, how?
- asked about red flag symptoms? If so, how long did this take? Was this sign-posted? (for example, did the doctor preface his questions with *"I need to ask some questions to rule out serious illness – do you have any of the following?"*)
- discussed the evidence base for appropriate treatments?
- provided appropriate occupational medicine advice?

If the consultation over-ran, did the doctor:

- take too long to ask the red flag questions?
- spend too much time on small-talk?
- attempt to reduce consulting time by offering the patient a face-to-face appointment instead? This option may not be the most efficient use of resources.

Revising data gathering

What questions could the doctor ask to discover the patient's ideas, concerns, expectations and health beliefs?

- Ideas: *"What, in your experience, has been the best way of dealing with food poisoning? What's worked, and not worked, for you in the past?"*
- Concerns: *"Is there anything in particular that concerns you about this positive campylobacter result?"*
- Expectations: *"It seems to me that we have discussed your symptoms and treatment. However, I suspect you may have some questions about work. There are any questions in particular you'd like me to answer?"*
- Health beliefs: *"You suspect that because this is your second episode of gut infection, you may be predisposed to gut infections. Let's talk about this for a moment."*

Test your theoretical knowledge

For each of the following statements, answer true (T) or false (F).

Regarding food poisoning

1. Diarrhoea, cramping, abdominal pain, and fever within 24 hours of exposure to the organism are symptoms of campylobacteriosis.
2. The absence of symptoms excludes a diagnosis of campylobacteriosis.
3. Campylobacteriosis is often associated with the consumption of seafood, soft cheese, or untreated water.
4. The source of campylobacteriosis is often not found.
5. Microbiological examination of faeces is useful if there is a suspected public health hazard, e.g. diarrhoea in food handlers and healthcare workers.

6. Microbiological examination of faeces is useful if the patient is systemically unwell or has dysentery.

7. Loperamide is useful and safe in people with severe symptoms or dysentery.

Relevant literature

http://cks.library.nhs.uk/mobiledevices/ckscontent.aspx?rawurl=gastroenteritis

http://cks.library.nhs.uk/gastroenteritis/background_information/causitive_infections/campylobacter

Case 14 – Man with UTI

Brief to the doctor

Mr MN is a 24 year old man attending for the result of a urine test taken a week previously by your nurse practitioner.

Patient summary

Name	MN
Date of birth (Age)	24
Social and family history	Single Engineer
Past medical history	1 week ago – Nurse Practitioner Clinic: "*4/7 dysuria, frequency and urgency. Urine Prot tr, WBC +, Nit Pos. Send MSU. Trimethoprim 200mg bd 7/7. Pt will call me in 4d for result.*"
Current medication	None

Investigations	1 week ago MSU:	
WBC	$>10^7$/ml	
RBC	Nil	
Scanty mixed growth	?significance	

Tasks for the doctor

In this case, the tasks are to:
- review the patient's response to treatment and relate this to the MSU result
- answer the patient's questions about how he developed a UTI

Brief to the patient – more about the patient

1. Profile:

- MN, a 24 year old engineering graduate, has worked for an international mining company since graduating 2 years ago
- shares a rented flat with his girlfriend, a nurse at the local hospital; they plan to get married next year and buy their own flat
- enjoys an active lifestyle and likes to keep fit and healthy
- he developed urinary symptoms just over a week ago, attended the nurse practitioner's minor illness clinic and was told he probably had a UTI. He was given a prescription for antibiotics and told to phone the nurse back for the result

2. He is seeing the doctor today because:

- he has some questions he would like to discuss, rather than phone as instructed:
  - he is concerned about how he developed a UTI
  - his symptoms have not changed with the antibiotics – does this mean the nurse got the diagnosis or treatment wrong?
- the frequency and urgency symptoms are causing a lot of disruption and embarrassment – he usually works on sites around the country and keeps having to find toilets in a hurry

3. Additional information:

- If the doctor asks specifically:
  - his work mates have teased him that he might have an STD. He has not noticed any symptoms. He has not had sex with anyone other than his girlfriend for the past 6 months. If he has an STD, does this mean his girlfriend has been unfaithful? His girlfriend is on the Pill; they do not use condoms.
  - while working in South Africa 8 months ago, he had unprotected sex with a secretary working in his company's offices in Cape Town. This continued over a 2 month period until he returned to the UK. He feels very guilty about this and has not told his girlfriend about it. Before returning to the UK, he went to a GU Medicine Clinic and had tests, including HIV, and was told he was clear.
- He wants the doctor to explain:
  - how UTIs are 'caught'
  - the MSU result
  - why the antibiotics given by the nurse practitioner have not worked
  - what other diagnoses are possible
  - whether other tests or treatments are required

- He had an episode of discharge when he was a student, but was treated and checked afterwards and told he was clear.
- If the doctor talks about HIV, Mr MN will want to discuss:
  - why another test is required as he was told he was clear in South Africa
  - the implications on insurance and getting a mortgage
  - the implications for his girlfriend and any children they might have
  - how and where the test will be done – he is concerned that someone at the hospital will recognise his name as he and his girlfriend know and socialise with a lot of the staff there
  - if the test was positive, how would the practice deal with this? Would staff be told about his status? How would the practice guarantee confidentiality?
  - if the test was positive, what treatment would he have to have and what are the success rates nowadays?
  - given his job travelling round the country and sometimes abroad, are there any restrictions or precautions he would have to take?
- If the doctor talks about chlamydia, Mr MN will want to discuss:
  - how it is caught
  - if he has it, does this mean his girlfriend has been unfaithful?
  - could the South African clinic have missed it?
  - if he caught it in South Africa, why has it only just started giving him symptoms, and why has his girlfriend not had any symptoms?
  - will his girlfriend need to be tested and how should he raise this with her?
- Mr MN prefers simple straightforward honest answers to questions and will repeat questions to the doctor if he feels the doctor is evading answering or not giving unequivocal answers. He would rather be told all the possibilities, however bad, than be kept in the dark.

Approach to be taken

A. Data gathering, examination and clinical assessment skills

1. Define the clinical problem: clarify why the patient has presented today
The doctor:
- reads the patient information provided prior to the consultation
- asks open questions to explore:
  - Mr MN's response to treatment – *"How are you getting on?"*
  - his concerns over why he has not improved – *"What do you make of that?"*
  - any other issues concerning him – *"Is there anything else you are worried this might be?"*
- empathises with Mr MN over the practical effects of his symptoms
- asks closed questions to clarify details about the symptoms, past history, and sexual history
- obtains a sexual history in order to assesses Mr MN's risk of HIV or STDs

2. Performs an appropriate physical or mental examination
- In this case, an examination is not required.

B. Clinical management skills

3. Make an appropriate working diagnosis
- The doctor, based on the history and MSU result should suspect chlamydia.
- This is a clinically sound hypothesis and is an appropriate use of probability.
- The doctor integrates information to raise the possibility of HIV.

4. Explain the problem to the patient using appropriate language
The doctor:
- having quickly established that Mr MN is intelligent and eager to understand his symptoms, addresses his agenda
- explains the MSU result and the possibility of chlamydia infection
- provides information on chlamydia, in particular, how it may be asymptomatic for some time
- explains that specific tests need to be done for chlamydia and that his girlfriend will need to be tested
- should adopt a patient-centred approach to ensure he addresses the patient's concerns and expectations
- uses chunking and checking information – *"Before I move on, can I check that I have got things clear?"*

5. *Provide holistic care and use resources effectively*
The doctor:
- practises evidence-based medicine – there is a likelihood of chlamydia given the MSU result, and a possibility of HIV given the history of unprotected sex in a high-risk country
- understands socioeconomic/cultural background – discusses ways of informing his girlfriend that she needs to be tested – *"Would you like to discuss how you might raise this matter with your girlfriend?"*
- is able to discuss the benefits and other implications of HIV testing – including insurance, mortgage, future health and travel
- provides Mr MN with verbal and written information on chlamydia and HIV

6. *Prescribe appropriately*
The doctor:
- advises Mr MN that a second HIV test is required before he can be told he is clear
- does not prescribe antibiotics as the diagnosis is not certain and other STDs must be excluded
- provides the patient with a referral letter to a GUM Clinic for investigation and consideration of HIV testing

7. *Specify the conditions and interval for follow-up*
The doctor:
- confirms understanding – *"Can I just check that I have explained things clearly – what is the plan for you?"*
- signposts Mr MN to information on chlamydia and HIV and to GUM Clinics where he could be tested
- offers a follow-up appointment to discuss any issues arising – safety netting

C. Interpersonal skills: know and treat this patient

8. *Achieve rapport*
The doctor:
- listens carefully to Mr MN's concerns about his symptoms not settling and the effects they have on him at work
- without embarrassment, sympathetically and sensitively elicits Mr MN's past sexual history
- places problem in psychosocial context – how it affects patient/girlfriend/work
- understands his request for information on chlamydia
- displays empathy when raising the question of whether Mr MN is at risk of HIV and should have another test
- helps Mr MN explore ways of raising the issues with his girlfriend – *"Would you like to practise how you might tell her?"*

- answers Mr MN's questions using appropriate language
- is non-judgemental about Mr MN's past sexual experiences
- addresses the patient's specific concerns and expectations – *"Is there anything else you want to ask me?"*

9. *Give the patient the opportunity to be involved in significant management decisions*
   The doctor:
   - actively confirms the patient's understanding of the problem – *"Does this make sense to you?"*
   - shares thoughts/involves patient – *"If I were to say that having unprotected sex in South Africa may have exposed you to HIV, what would you say?"*
   - agrees balanced plans – *"Are you happy with this plan?"*

Debrief

This starts as a relatively straightforward clinical case; the real challenge is communication skills with the patient over the possibility of chlamydia, how he could have caught it and the implications on his relationship, and finally the issue of HIV. The ability to take a sexual history without being awkward or embarrassed is also tested.

Discuss how the doctor could, if needed, improve his performance. In particular, assess how the doctor:
- answered questions in language and style that satisfied Mr MN
- discussed the sensitive issues of infidelity, STDs and HIV
- developed empathy and trust
- managed time in the consultation – not wasting time gathering information at the expense of discussing the sensitive issues

Revising data gathering

What questions could the doctor ask to discover the patient's ideas, concerns, expectations and health beliefs?
- Ideas: *"You said that work colleagues have teased you about having an STD, could that be a possibility?"*
- Concerns: *"Would you like to discuss how chlamydia is caught and the range of symptoms it can cause?"*
- Expectations: *"The result of your urine test has not proven a normal infection; have you considered other possible causes?"*
- Health beliefs: *"You seem concerned that I am suggesting another HIV test even though you were given the 'all-clear' in South Africa, shall we talk about HIV testing?"*

Once the doctor has gathered sufficient information, how could he summarise the problem for the patient?
- Evaluate whether the doctor used appropriate language, paced his explanation, and whether the explanation was well organised and logical.

Test your theoretical knowledge

For each of the following statements, answer true (T) or false (F)
1. Approximately 20% of females infected with chlamydia are asymptomatic
2. *N. gonorrhoeaea* and *Chlamydia trachomatis* account for most cases of epididymitis in men under 35 years of age
3. Bacterial orchitis rarely occurs with an associated epididymitis and is usually bilateral
4. Untreated neonatal chlamydia conjunctivitis can result in blindness

5. A significant percentage of men and women with gonorrhoea also have pharyngitis, which is usually asymptomatic

Relevant literature

Rogstad KE, Palfreeman A, Rooney G, *et al.* (2006) *United Kingdom national guidelines on HIV testing.* London: Clinical Effectiveness Group, British Association of Sexual Health and HIV.

Chlamydia: www.emedicine.com/emerg/TOPIC925.HTM

Gonorrhoea: www.emedicine.com/emerg/TOPIC220.HTM

Orchitis: www.emedicine.com/emerg/TOPIC344.HTM

Case 15 – Childhood bedwetting

Brief to the doctor

Mrs DJ is a 29 year old woman who presents (without her 6 year old son) asking for advice on his bedwetting.

Patient summary

Name	Tomas J
Date of birth (Age)	6
Social and Family History	One sister, age 3
Past medical history	Healthy – achieved appropriate milestones for age Seen occasionally for mild, seasonal URTIs
Repeat medication	None

Tasks for the doctor

In this case, the tasks are to:
- clarify the extent and nature of the bedwetting
- the effect of the bedwetting on Tomas and his family
- provide evidence-based advice on treatments

Brief to the patient – more about the patient

1. Profile:

- Mrs DJ is 29 year old housewife; her husband is a car mechanic
- both her children are healthy and developing as expected
- Mrs DJ is worried about her 6 year old son's bedwetting

2. She is seeing the doctor today because:

- she is concerned that Tomas still wets the bed at least 2 times per week. He has never been dry at night, but he is dry during the day. He has no medical problems and does not suffer from constipation or urine infections.
- he is a lovely child who is achieving well at school; he has lots of friends
- she has declined the sleep-overs to which Tomas has been invited as she thinks it would be embarrassing for him if he bed-wets on a sleepover – she worries about him being teased
- now that her daughter is 3, she would like to leave her children with her mum for a week so that she and her husband can go on holiday, but the frequent changing and washing of bedding creates a burden of housework and she feels guilty approaching her 56 year old mother
- nobody in the family has had a bedwetting problem
- she has tried restricting drinks for Tomas at night but this has not made much difference
- she thought the problem would resolve by age 5, but Tomas is now 6. Does he have a problem predisposing him to bedwetting? Should he be investigated? Does he need tablet treatments? Is there anything else she should do?

3. Additional information:

- if the doctor refers her to the health visitor, she would like to know what she should expect in terms of assessment and advice?
- if the doctor mentions different options to her, she expects to be advised on the efficacy of each before deciding on what she would like for Tomas

Approach to be taken

A. Data gathering, examination and clinical assessment skills

1. Define the clinical problem: clarify why the patient has presented today
The doctor:
- notes from the patient information provided that this is a 6 year old with no significant past medical history
- asks mum open questions to explore the nature of the bedwetting (to make a diagnosis of primary nocturnal enuresis in a healthy, socially well adjusted 6 year old boy)
- asks what has made her present today (to discover that Mrs DJ is thinking of leaving the children with her mum for a week in the school holidays to have a break with her husband)
- asks closed questions to identify potentially reversible contributory factors: constipation, urinary tract infections, diet, stress (school problems / family discord / moving house), diabetes mellitus, ease of access to a toilet or potty, night lights, and bunk beds
- excludes red flags: neurological problems, behaviour problems, sleep apnoea
- elicits how the problem affects Tomas (embarrassment, social isolation, teasing by family members or friends)
- elicits how the problem affects the family (parental anxiety / frustration / punishment / extra work of laundry / effect of interrupted sleep)
- discovers her ideas that bedwetting should have ceased by age 6
- discovers her concerns about the social restriction (sleep-overs / family holidays)
- discovers her expectations for advice and a treatment plan

2. Performs an appropriate physical or mental examination
- In this case, an examination is not required. However, make arrangements to examine Tomas (abdomen, genitalia, spine (tuft of hair/lipoma), knee jerks, and a dipstick urinalysis).

B. Clinical management skills

3. Make an appropriate working diagnosis
- The doctor, based on the history, makes a working diagnosis of childhood primary nocturnal enuresis. There are no contributory factors.

4. Explain the problem to the patient using appropriate language
The doctor:
- contextualises the problem: 1 in 50 7 year olds wet the bed more than once a week and 15% get better without treatment each year. Children who are passing large volumes at night may not be producing sufficient

anti-diuretic hormone (ADH); small volumes may indicate small, irritable bladders; or the child may be sleeping so deeply that he is unaware of the sensation of a full bladder.

- having established the absence of red flags and contributory factors, provides general support and advice: signposting to ERIC (enuresis resource and information centre), using waterproof mattress coverings, avoiding caffeine after 3 pm, timing and amount of fluid intake
- refers to the health visitor for specific advice: star charts to reward getting out of bed to use the toilet, or enuresis alarms (bed or body-worn) for the child to learn to stop urinating when the alarm sounds – because they require the child's cooperation, alarms are usually reserved for children over 7 years
- advises Mrs DJ that drug treatment, with imipramine or desmopressin, is appropriate for short periods such a sleep-overs or holidays away from home; both drugs can be used in a 6 year old, and are effective while taken but bedwetting recurs on discontinuation

5. *Provide holistic care and use resources effectively*
   The doctor:
   - practises evidence-based medicine that is informed by national or local guidelines (www.cks.library.nhs.uk/enuresis_nocturnal/view_whole_topic)
   - involves the health visitor in on-going treatment and support
   - does not refer to secondary care in the absence of red flags and contributory symptoms

6. *Prescribe appropriately*
   The doctor:
   - is aware of the indications and side-effects of imipramine and desmopressin
   - discusses prescription but is unlikely to prescribe without having examined the child and organised urine tests first

7. *Specify the conditions and interval for follow-up*
   The doctor:
   - signposts Mrs DJ to information on nocturnal enuresis, such as www.eric.org.uk/
   - arranges urinalysis
   - offers a follow-up appointment to examine Tomas, discuss urine test findings, and review the problem

C. Interpersonal skills: know and treat this patient

8. *Achieve rapport*
   The doctor:
   - listens attentively to Mrs DJ's concerns regarding the continued bedwetting and its impact on the family
   - displays empathy to the workload and financial burden the bedwetting creates
   - addresses the patient's specific expectations about a long-term solution and what to do for sleep-overs and holidays
   - is sensitive in his queries regarding the parents' frustration and the possible punishment of the child

9. *Give the patient the opportunity to be involved in significant management decisions*
   The doctor:
   - shares his thoughts, for example, *"I am reassured by what you have told me about Tomas's physical and social development. I think this problem will resolve in time as his hormones and bladder mature. There are a few things we could do to help Tomas. I'll give you the options first and then you can tell me which you'd like to try."*
   - encourages autonomy and opinions – provides her with information so she feels able to choose the most appropriate option for Tomas and the family

Debrief

Discuss how the doctor could, if needed, improve his performance. In particular, assess whether the doctor:

- structured the history taking? For example, did the doctor preface his questions with *"I need to ask some questions to rule out serious illness – does Tomas have any of the following?"*
- assessed the impact of the bedwetting on the entire family? If so, how?
- addressed Mrs DJ's specific concerns? If so, how?
- made appropriate use of resources?
- outlined the reasons for follow-up?

If the consultation over-ran, did the doctor:

- ask open rather than closed questions when assessing contributory and red flag symptoms?
- provide overly detailed explanations of each option?
- signpost inadequately, that is, duplicate the services of the health visitor (or continence advisor) in providing detailed information and on-going support?

Revising data gathering

What questions could the doctor ask to discover the patient's ideas, concerns, expectations and health beliefs?

- Ideas: *"What is your understanding of bedwetting – causes, treatments and so on?"*
- Concerns: *"Is there anything in particular about the current situation that is worrying you?"*
- Expectations: *"When you came to see me today, was there anything in particular you'd hoped I'd do for you?"*
- Health beliefs: *"You seem concerned that your 6 year old hasn't achieved night-time dryness. Let's talk about this for a moment."*

Test your theoretical knowledge

For each of the following statements, answer true (T) or false (F).

Regarding childhood nocturnal enuresis

1. Enuresis is the involuntary discharge of urine by day or night or both, in a child aged 6 years or older, in the absence of congenital or acquired defects of the nervous system or urinary tract.
2. Up to one-third of parents become intolerant of the enuresis and consequently also of their child.
3. 10% of children with nocturnal enuresis have a positive family history of childhood bedwetting.
4. The treatment of chronic constipation leads to the resolution of nocturnal enuresis in two-thirds of affected children.

5. The odds ratio of enuresis in children with ADHD is 2.7 times higher than in controls.
6. Cola and chocolate are diuretics.
7. The only investigation required in primary nocturnal enuresis is urinalysis to exclude diabetes mellitus and a urinary tract infection.
8. Restrict fluids such that the child has about six small drinks a day, spaced out throughout the day, the last one 2 hours before bed.
9. Sharing a room is a relative contra-indication to the use of an enuresis alarm.
10. Desmopressin and imipramine are of equal efficacy.

Relevant literature

www.cks.library.nhs.uk/enuresis_nocturnal/view_whole_topic

Case 16 – Prostate cancer

Brief to the doctor

Mr OP is a 74 year old man who saw a locum 4 days ago because of urinary symptoms. The locum arranged tests for MSU, FBC, U&Es, LFTs and PSA. Mr OP attends today for the results.

Patient summary

Name	OP
Date of birth (Age)	74
Social and family history	Married Retired carpenter and joiner No FH CVD
Past medical history	4 days ago – Locum: *"Frequency, nocturia x4, dribbling. Urine NAD. Abdo NAD. RE hard nodular left lobe prostate. Check bloods and review prior to referral. Pt not told prostate feels suspicious."*
Current medication	None

Investigations	4 days ago:
Hb	11.2 g/dl (12–15)
MCV	78.4 (83–105)
WBC	2.3 (4–11)
ESR	84
Na	130 (135–145)
K	3.4 (3.5–5)
Urea	5.6 (2.5–6.7)
Creatinine	76 (70–150)
AlkP	185 (95–280)
AST	28
ALT	31 (10–45)
PSA	10 (<4.0)

Tasks for the doctor

In this case, the tasks are to:
- review results and the locum's clinical findings
- explain the results and the necessary actions to the patient
- deal with the patient's anxiety over the possible diagnosis

Brief to the patient – more about the patient

1. Profile:

- Mr OP is a 74 year old retired carpenter and joiner
- he likes to keeps active, although after a hip replacement 4 years ago he has not been as active as he hoped he would be
- he has been troubled with increasing frequency, nocturia and dribbling stream for the past year, but things have got worse over the past 2 months
- he feels well in himself, but gets tired easily – he attributes this to his age
- he does not like to make a fuss and believes doctors should not be questioned – they are experts and he should take their advice

2. He is seeing the doctor today because:

- the locum doctor took some tests and told him to come back to see one of the regular doctors for the results
- a lot of his friends have prostate problems and are taking tablets that help; he expects the doctor is going to start him on these today

3. Additional information:

- If the doctor asks specifically:
  - symptoms – nocturia x4, frequency by day every 60–90 minutes, weak stream with terminal dribbling; no blood seen
  - he has not lost any weight and has no other symptoms
  - his father's brother died of prostate cancer. His father died of old age. His uncle was treated by orchidectomy – Mr OP is horrified at this treatment.
- If the doctor suggests that the results are suspicious or that referral for more tests is required, Mr OP will ask if there is a possibility of cancer.
- He is still sexually active.
- His wife had a small heart attack 2 years ago, but is well and active now. He tries not to trouble her with things because she is a worrier and he is concerned that worrying will strain her heart.
- He has two children who both live locally and visit regularly.
- He has not considered the possibility of having cancer because he feels well, unlike his uncle who was ill and lost a lot of weight.
- If the doctor mentions cancer:
  - he will get very anxious about his wife, possible treatments and prognosis
  - he will want the doctor to explain what treatments are possible and their success
  - he will want to discuss what he should tell his wife and whether it will affect her heart

Approach to be taken

A. Data gathering, examination and clinical assessment skills

1. *Define the clinical problem: clarify why the patient has presented today*
The doctor:
- reads the patient information provided prior to the consultation
- asks open questions to explore what the locum told Mr OP and what Mr OP suspects might be the cause of his symptoms: "*Can you tell me what the locum said to you?*" and "*What do you think might be the cause?*"
- asks closed questions to clarify Mr OP's symptoms and family history
- responds to non-verbal cues: "*You look like you weren't expecting to be told you needed to be referred, am I right?*"

2. *Performs an appropriate physical or mental examination*
- In this case, an examination is not required.

B. Clinical management skills

3. *Make an appropriate working diagnosis*
- The doctor integrates information from the history, the locum's examination and blood results and makes a working diagnosis of suspected prostatic cancer.

4. *Explain the problem to the patient using appropriate language*
The doctor:
- informs Mr OP that the blood test results and the locum's examination are not normal and that further tests at the hospital are indicated
- uses a patient-centred approach to address Mr OP's concerns and expectations – "*I cannot say whether this is cancer or not until you have had some tests at the hospital*"
- checks the patient's understanding: "*This has been a bit of a shock for you, can I just go over what we have just talked about before moving on to the next bit?*"
- provides some information on what tests may be required, and what treatments are available: transrectal ultrasound, biopsy, bone scans, treatments depend on stage and assessed risk and range from active surveillance only through surgery to radiotherapy and chemo- and hormone therapy

5. *Provide holistic care and use resources effectively*
The doctor:
- practises evidence-based medicine and is informed by national or local guidelines – NICE (2008) *Prostate cancer: diagnosis and treatment*

- allows Mr OP time to explore his anxieties about telling his wife his possible diagnosis
- provides Mr OP with information if required

6. *Prescribe appropriately*
The doctor:
- is aware of national and local guidelines:
  - for suspected cancer referrals: NICE (2005) *Referral guidelines for suspected cancer* (CG27 – www.nice.org.uk/Guidance/CG27)
  - for prostate cancer: NICE (2008) *Prostate cancer: diagnosis and treatment* (CG58 – www.nice.org.uk/Guidance/CG58)

7. *Specify the conditions and interval for follow-up*
The doctor:
- offers a follow-up appointment to discuss any issues arising from his outpatient attendance or if Mr OP has any questions or concerns
- safety netting – "*You should have received an appointment to be seen within the next 2 weeks; let me know if you have heard nothing in one week's time*"
- arranges to see Mr OP after the hospital appointment

C. Interpersonal skills: know and treat this patient

8. *Achieve rapport*
The doctor:
- sensitively informs Mr OP about the need for referral
- explores and clarifies Mr OP's concerns and expectations: "*You look concerned. Is there anything particular worrying you?*"
- listens attentively to Mr OP's concerns about his wife
- displays empathy: "*I understand why you are worried about the effect this might have on your wife; would you like to discuss this for a while?*"

9. *Give the patient the opportunity to be involved in significant management decisions*
The doctor:
- actively confirms the patient's understanding of the problem: "*What does all this mean to you?*"
- provides the patient with information by answering his questions, but does not raise unnecessary alarm as the diagnosis has not been confirmed
- supports the patient by discussing his concerns about possible treatments (particularly orchidectomy) and how to tell his wife

Debrief

This case focuses on the doctor's ability to raise the possibility of bad news.

Discuss how the doctor could, if needed, improve his performance. In particular, assess how the doctor:
- managed time in the consultation – did s/he spend too much time reviewing symptoms and not enough on answering Mr OP's concerns?
- raised the need for further tests and answered Mr OP's question about whether or not he had cancer

Revising data gathering

What questions could the doctor ask to discover the patient's ideas, concerns, expectations and health beliefs?
- Ideas: "*I understand that you wouldn't want the same treatment your uncle had; do you know anything about other treatments?*"
- Concerns: "*I understand that cancer is a frightening word, would you like to discuss prostate cancer in more detail?*"
- Expectations: "*I am going to refer you to the hospital; would you like me to outline what tests they are likely to want to do?*"
- Health beliefs: "*You are worried that this might affect your wife's health; would you like to spend some time talking about this?*"

Test your theoretical knowledge

For each of the following statements, answer true (T) or false (F).
1. Serum PSA level alone is a poor predictor of the presence of prostate cancer
2. Risk factors include diets high in red meats and fat
3. An affected first degree relative triples the relative risk
4. In low risk men, radical treatment may be deferred until there is evidence of progression of the cancer
5. Hormonal therapy is routinely offered to all men with intermediate or high risk of localised prostate cancer

Relevant literature

UK Prostate Link: www.prostate-link.org.uk

Cancer Research UK: www.cancerresearchuk.org

A framework for breaking bad news: www.skillscascade.com/badnews

DoH (2003) Breaking Bad News... Regional Guidelines. *Department of Health, Social Services and Public Safety, Northern Ireland Group of the National Council for Hospice and Specialist Palliative care*: www.dhsspni.gov.uk

Fallon M. (1998) ABC of palliative care: Communication with patients, families and other professionals. *BMJ*, **316**: 130–132.

Maguir GP. (1999) Breaking bad news: explaining cancer diagnosis and prognosis. *MJA*, **171**: 288–289.

Case 17 - Painful calf

Brief to the doctor

Mrs RD is a 29 year old woman who presents with a painful left calf.

Patient summary

Name	RD
Date of birth (Age)	29
Social and Family History	Married, no children Teacher Non-smoker
Past medical history	Difficulty sleeping (1 year ago) – given zopiclone Cervical smear 5 years ago – normal
Repeat medication	None
Tests	Values are from 6 months ago
BMI	24.2
BP	118/72
	Value from 1 year ago
PHQ score	6/27

Tasks for the doctor

In this case, the tasks are to:
- clarify whether Mrs RD's fears about having a DVT are well-founded
- negotiate appropriate and timely investigation
- explain the nature of the investigation(s) in simple, jargon-free language

Brief to the patient – more about the patient

1. Profile:

- Mrs RD is a 29 year old woman who works as a teacher in the local primary school
- when she married 4 months ago, she stopped taking the combined oral contraceptive pill (Microgynon) which she had used, without problems, since the age of 19; she hopes to get pregnant and her period is 2 days late – she has not done a pregnancy test as yet

2. She is seeing the doctor today because:

- her left calf has been painful for 36 hours – it feels swollen and warm to the touch
- she drove down from Edinburgh to London 3 days ago; there were problems on the road and the journey took 11 hours, but there was no opportunity during the 3 hour delay to leave the car
- she does not have a past history of deep vein thrombosis (DVT), is no longer on Microgynon, and has not had recent surgery. Her sister (aged 28) had a DVT during the 20th week of her pregnancy. Nobody else in the family has had a DVT or pulmonary embolus (PE).
- she has not done any recent strenuous physical exercise, nor does she feel unwell in herself

3. Additional information:

- Mrs RD is worried that she may be pregnant and she may have a DVT
- she expects a referral to the hospital for a scan
- her sister was given injections to treat the DVT – will she be put on injections too? She has needle-phobia and does not believe that she will manage to self-inject.

Approach to be taken

A. Data gathering, examination and clinical assessment skills

1. *Define the clinical problem: clarify why the patient has presented today*
   The doctor:
   - reads the patient information provided prior to the consultation
   - asks open questions to explore the nature and duration of the symptoms
   - empathises with Mrs RD's concerns that this may be a DVT
   - asks closed questions to assess whether the patient is at high risk for DVT: previous history of DVT, recent surgery, recent immobility, malignancy?
   - asks about PE symptoms: shortness or breath, pleuritic chest pain, haemoptysis?
   - works through the diagnostic sieve to rule out other possible causes of a painful calf, such as cellulitis, lymphangitis, muscle strain, a ruptured Baker's cyst, or venous insufficiency. The doctor could sign-post his systematic questioning of the differential diagnosis by prefacing his questions with: *"I need to ask some questions to rule out all the possible causes of a sore calf – do you have any of the following symptoms: a red rash on the calf, feeling unwell in yourself, muscle strain from sport or an injury?"*.
   - asks about the possibility of pregnancy, an important red flag
   - discovers Mrs RD's idea that she has a DVT, her concern that she will need to treat the DVT by self injecting, her expectation of a referral to hospital for a scan and her belief that DVTs are treated by subcutaneous heparin

2. *Performs an appropriate physical or mental examination*
   - An examination is required and should be guided by the Wells scoring system – see www.wolg.org.uk/DVTblank.rtf or www.pulsetoday.co.uk/ Journals/Medical/Pulse/2008_April_23/attachments/Wells%20DVT%20 scoring.pdf
   - Look for:
     - tenderness along entire deep vein system
     - swelling of entire leg
     - measure the calf circumference 10 cm below the tibial tuberosity and look for >3 cm difference in calf circumference
     - pitting oedema confined to the symptomatic leg
     - collateral dilated superficial veins (non-varicose)
     - the absence of signs pointing to an alternative diagnosis, such as cellulitis, congestive cardiac failure, muscle sprains or a Baker's cyst
   - In this patient, assume the only sign present is moderate tenderness (4/10) in the posterior aspect of the left calf which is worse when the patient stands up or when you passively dorsiflex her ankle.

B. Clinical management skills

3. *Make an appropriate working diagnosis*
   - The doctor, based on the history and examination, makes a working diagnosis of DVT. If the patient is not pregnant, the risk is low and a D-dimer test should be done. If the patient is pregnant, the risk is moderate to high and an ultrasound scan should be organised.

4. *Explain the problem to the patient using appropriate language*
   The doctor:
   - having clarified that Mrs RD has a good idea of what a DVT is based on her sister's experience, addresses her agenda
   - explains that further investigation (blood test or ultrasound scan) depends on whether or not she is pregnant – the doctor organises a pregnancy test
   - addresses her idea that she has a DVT. She may have a DVT, but further investigation is needed before a diagnosis can be made. Only 50% of patients with classic signs of a DVT actually have one.
   - Addresses her concerns: she is worried about self-injecting subcutaneous heparin. If she is pregnant and has a DVT (two assumptions at present), subcutaneous heparin is needed. If she is not pregnant and has a DVT, a brief period of subcutaneous injection is followed by oral wafarin therapy. The fact that injections are subcuteous (rather than intramuscular) and may only be needed for a brief period may be reassuring to the patient.
   - Addresses her expectations: a scan is needed only if her pregnancy test is positive, or if her D-dimer result is positive.

5. *Provide holistic care and use resources effectively*
   The doctor:
   - practises evidence-based medicine
   - is informed by national or local guidelines (http://cks.library.nhs.uk/deep_vein_thrombosis/management)

6. *Prescribe appropriately*
   The doctor:
   - is aware of national and local guidelines
   - does not prescribe until further information is available

7. *Specify the conditions and interval for follow-up*
   The doctor:
   - arranges for a pregnancy test. If positive, arranges for a scan. If negative, arranges for a D-dimer test.
   - if DVT is suspected on clinical grounds, further assessment and definitive diagnosis on the day of presentation is ideal

C. Interpersonal skills: know and treat this patient

8. *Achieve rapport*
   The doctor:
   - listens attentively to Mrs RD's concerns about having a DVT
   - understands her request for an ultrasound scan and deals with the request appropriately and with sensitivity
   - gently challenges or corrects the patient's assumption that she has a DVT requiring treatment with subcutaneous heparin

9. *Give the patient the opportunity to be involved in significant management decisions*
   The doctor:
   - negotiates with the patient when the pregnancy test will be done
   - gives the patient sufficient information to appreciate that time is of the essence and definitive testing should be completed within 24 hours of presentation

Debrief

Discuss how the doctor could, if needed, improve his performance. In particular, assess whether the doctor:

- took a systematic history, quickly eliciting the risk factors for DVT, and working through the diagnostic sieve
- discussed and prioritised the order of the investigations, while addressing the patient's expectation of a scan appropriately
- explained the investigations (D-dimer testing) in simple language

If the consultation over-ran, was the doctor:

- systematic in his history taking – were questions asked without appropriate signposting?
- systematic, thorough and confident in his examination technique?
- logical and organised in arranging further investigation and follow-up?

Revising data gathering

What questions could the doctor ask to discover the patient's ideas, concerns, expectations and health beliefs?

- Ideas: *"What, do you imagine, the treatment for DVT will be?"*
- Concerns: *"With regard to DVTs, what are you most worried about?"*
- Expectations: *"How was your sister's DVT diagnosed? Did you also expect to be scanned?"*
- Health beliefs: *"You have good grounds for suspecting a DVT. Let's just talk about how we go about confirming or disproving a DVT."*

Test your theoretical knowledge

For each of the following statements, answer true (T) or false (F).

Regarding DVT and PE

1. Dyspnoea, chest pain, or haemoptysis are symptoms of DVT.
2. A positive Homan's sign is pain in the calf on active abrupt, forceful dorsiflexion of the ankle with the leg outstretched (knee extended).
3. The D-dimer assay is a test for the presence of fibrin degradation products in plasma, which are raised in DVT.
4. Pregnancy raises plasma levels of D-dimer.
5. D-dimer assays are less sensitive for proximal than distal DVT.
6. D-dimer levels are unaffected by heparin.
7. Moderate to high risk patients, with a positive D-dimer test and a negative ultrasound, do not require repeat ultrasonography.
8. One of the differential diagnoses of a DVT is a ruptured Baker's cyst, which is a cyst that forms in the ankle from an outpouching of synovial membrane of the ankle joint.

Relevant literature

http://cks.library.nhs.uk/deep_vein_thrombosis/management

www.youtube.com/watch?v=Y2XHP-aaDpc – presentation on DVT by Stephen Bright

www.bcshguidelines.com/pdf/OutpatientDVT_211003.pdf

Case 18 – Leg ulcer

Brief to the doctor

Miss QR is an 85 year old lady who is usually seen regularly in surgery by your senior partner (Dr Smith). She has requested a home visit because she has knocked her leg and it is 'leaking water'.

Patient summary

Name	QR
Date of birth (Age)	85
Social and family history	Lives alone in privately owned old people's flat Warden on site
Past medical history	Hypertension – 30 years Leg oedema – 4 years Osteoarthritis both knees – 15 years Obesity – 45 years
	Saw Dr Smith 1 month ago: "*No great change. BP 140/84, oedema to just above knees. Walking with a stick. Blood test done. No change in medication.*"
Current medication	Lisinopril 20 mg daily Furosemide 40 mg twice daily
Investigations	1 month ago – FBC, U&Es and fasting glucose all normal

Tasks for the doctor

In this case, the tasks are to:
- explore and clarify Miss QR's concerns
- formulate an appropriate clinical and social management plan, utilising other members of the PCT

Brief to the patient – more about the patient

1. Profile:

- Miss QR is an 85 year old lady who lives alone in a privately owned old flat in an old peoples' block with a resident warden
- she has long-standing hypertension and osteoarthritis in her knees. She has been overweight most of her life and knows she should lose weight, but has no motivation to do so. For the past 4 years her legs have been swollen and this is limiting her mobility significantly.
- she attends surgery every 3 months for a check with Dr Smith
- she has no family history of CVD or DM

2. She is seeing the doctor today because:

- she knocked her leg on the corner of a coffee table last week, causing a superficial wound which she put a plaster on initially, but she started to leak fluid from the wound and when she removed the plaster she tore off skin, leaving a superficial raw area
- the leg has continued to leak. Friends have bought dressings and bandages from the local chemist who has now suggested to them that she should be seen. She has to sit with plastic bags under her leg to prevent the carpet getting soiled and has had to put a waterproof mattress cover on her bed. She is very meticulous about hygiene and finds the leaking fluid repugnant.
- she is terrified of developing leg ulcers
- she is very proud that her blood tests for kidney function, diabetes and cholesterol have always been normal and feels that this justifies her belief that there would be no real benefit to her if she lost weight
- she feels well despite the current problem

3. Additional information:

- If the doctor asks specifically:
  - she lives on the first floor, but there is a lift
  - she has been elevating her legs on a low stool
- She will not accept hospital admission unless she is very ill.
- She has a home help who visits once weekly to clean and do her shopping. Miss QR can cook for herself and is completely independent.
- She believes a District Nurse should be asked to visit and dress her leg.
- She is struggling to cope with her single stick and believes a frame might be a better option; she is reluctant to ask for this as she feels she is being over-demanding when resources in the NHS are scarce.
- If the doctor examines her:

System	Examination findings
General	No pallor. Grossly overweight.
CVS	HR 76 SR. HS 1+2 +nil. BP 136/82 Lungs clear Pitting oedema to mid-thigh level Unable to palpate pedal pulses due to oedema
Abdo	No mass. No organomegaly. No ascites.
Legs	Oedema as noted OA knees with valgus deformity on right 4×4cm superficial ulcer left shin. Very thin shiny surrounding skin with some small scattered vesicles. No surrounding cellulitis and no slough on ulcer. No evidence of infection. Serous fluid leaking from ulcer.

Approach to be taken

A. Data gathering, examination and clinical assessment skills

1. *Define the clinical problem: clarify why the patient has presented today*
   The doctor:
   - reads the patient information provided prior to the consultation
   - asks open questions to explore why she has asked for a home visit a week after injuring her leg – *"Have you any thoughts about what can be done to help you?"*
   - empathises with her about the leaking fluid
   - asks closed questions to clarify details about her past history and current medication, and her general health at present

2. *Performs an appropriate physical or mental examination*
   - Explains that an examination is required using appropriate language.
   - Performs a targeted examination to assess wound and degree of heart failure – this should include looking at the wound, assessing the extent of her oedema, checking JVP and listening to her heart and lungs.
   - Examination addresses patient's concerns – to see whether she has an ulcer.

B. Clinical management skills

3. *Make an appropriate working diagnosis*
   - The doctor, based on the history and examination, makes a working diagnosis of leg ulcer in a lady with heart failure.

4. *Explain the problem to the patient using appropriate language*
   The doctor:
   - explains why the ulcer has developed and why it has continued to leak fluid
   - addresses the patient's concerns and expectations – *"There is a good chance we can get the ulcer to heal as it is shallow, but we will need to decrease your leg swelling to help this happen."*

5. *Provide holistic care and use resources effectively*
   The doctor:
   - arranges for the District Nurse to visit to assess the ulcer and provide appropriate dressings and monitor response
   - explains what the District Nurse is likely to do – Doppler Ankle Brachial Pressure Index (ABPI)
   - provides some information on what Miss QR can do to help herself – good skin care, low salt intake, importance of mobility and exercise, leg elevation when immobile
   - identifies the social (decreased mobility) and psychological (finds the leaking fluid repugnant) impact of this diagnosis on Miss QR

- uses PCT and other resources – District Nurse and physiotherapy/OT assessment of whether a frame might enable safer mobility than her current stick

6. *Prescribe appropriately*
The doctor:
- decides to see if rest and elevation will be beneficial before altering treatment
- decides to await the result of the ABPI before formulating an ulcer management plan

7. *Specify the conditions and interval for follow-up*
The doctor:
- offers a follow-up appointment either with him/herself or with Dr Smith to monitor progress
- confirms understanding – *"Is there anything I haven't explained or you don't understand?"*

C. Interpersonal skills: know and treat this patient

8. *Achieve rapport*
The doctor:
- explores and clarifies Miss QR's concerns – *"Is there anything in particular you are worried about?"*
- places problem in psychosocial context – *"How are you coping with all this on your own?"*
- supports the long relationship Miss QR has with Dr Smith
- addresses the patient's specific concerns and expectations – District Nurse visit and provision of a frame

9. *Give the patient the opportunity to be involved in significant management decisions*
The doctor:
- actively confirms patient's understanding of the problem – *"Have I adequately explained to you why your leg is leaking fluid?"*
- uses time as a therapeutic tool – no medication change, monitor effects of ulcer treatment and elevation
- encourages autonomy and opinions – *"Have you had any thoughts on what I can do to help?"*
- supports and congratulates her in looking after the ulcer initially and preventing infection

Debrief

Discuss how the doctor could, if needed, improve his performance. In particular, assess how the doctor:
- established rapport with a patient who usually saw another doctor
- explored Miss QR's concerns and beliefs
- explained the possible management plans that may result from the ABPI results

Revising data gathering

What questions could the doctor ask to discover the patient's ideas, concerns, expectations and health beliefs?
- Ideas: *"Why do you think the wound has not healed as quickly as you expected?"*
- Concerns: *"Is there anything you are particularly worried about?"*
- Expectations: *"You have done really well to keep the wound clean, but it isn't healing as you expected. What do you think needs to be done now?"*
- Health beliefs: *"The pharmacist advised getting the wound checked – let's discuss wound healing briefly."*

Test your theoretical knowledge

For each of the following statements, answer true (T) or false (F).
1. The cause of most leg ulcers is unclear
2. A past history of cigarette smoking, phlebitis and previous trauma should always be taken
3. Skin pigmentation, shiny hairless skin and varicose veins suggest an arterial cause
4. ABPI measurements in patients with diabetes may not be reliable
5. Ulcers should be scrubbed clean to remove all debris and exudate
6. Graduated compression bandages should be used to control oedema
7. Patients with an ABPI <0.5 require urgent referral
8. Ulcers should be swabbed routinely so that any infection can be identified and treated promptly

Relevant literature

www.sign.ac.uk/pdf/sign26.pdf

www.worldwidewounds.com/2001/march/Vowdenb/Doppler-asssessment-and-ABPI

http://clinicalevidence.bmj.com/ceweb/conditions/wnd/1902/1902_background.jsp

Case 19 – A list of symptoms

Brief to the doctor

Mrs SW is a 52 year old woman who presents with a list of problems:
1. pain in right calf
2. voice is hoarse
3. I had recent blood tests – what are the results
4. I think I'm going through the menopause – feeling low, tired, no sex drive, weight gain

Patient summary

Name	SW
Date of birth (Age)	52
Social and Family History	Married for 28 years with one child (27) Works from home providing IT support
Past medical history	Sleep disorders (8 months ago) – issued zopiclone Right leg sciatica (8 months ago) – issued analgesia Voice hoarseness (3 years ago) – no abnormalities found by ENT; assumed related to gastric reflux Intermittent asthma (from teenager)
Repeat medication	Diprobase 500 g as directed (AD) Seretide 125 evohaler Cfc-free 100 µg / puff (AD) Ventolin evohaler Cfc-free 100 µg / puff (AD) Lansoprazole 30 mg once daily x 28

Consultation note by Dr Brown (4 weeks ago):
'Voice hoarseness: has had previous episodes and investigations by ENT in the past. No evidence of cancer and felt related to gastric reflux. Gargles after using steroid inhalers. Has been having more reflux symptoms lately despite cutting down alcohol dramatically from 50 units per week and changing diet. Last week, only had 4 glasses of wine in total. O/E: no cervical lymph nodes felt. Throat OK. Chest clear. No creps or wheeze. Plan: Trial of doubling PPI. Get bloods for general health screen. Review thereafter.'

Blood tests	Tests were done two weeks ago
Hb	12.5 g/dl (12–15)
MCV	102 (83–105)
Liver functions tests	normal
Renal function	normal
TSH	4.32 (0.35–5.5)
Fasting glucose	6.2 (3–5.5)
Total cholesterol	5.7
HDL	1.1
H. pylori	negative

Tasks for the doctor

In this case, the tasks are to:
- negotiate the problem list, prioritising appropriately
- discuss the blood results, especially the abnormal fasting glucose
- discuss the menopausal symptoms
- establish that the calf pain and hoarse voice are long-standing problems, without recent red-flags, and agree review of these issues at follow-up appointments

Brief to the patient – more about the patient

1. Profile:

- Mrs SW is a 52 year old woman who has worked from home for the last 6 months. She misses the social interaction of working in an office environment and now feels lonely and low.
- she is happily married; her husband has noticed the increased alcohol consumption, which she has attributed to helping her sleep at night
- Mrs SW doesn't see the doctor often and because she is worried about her health, she presents with a list of symptoms. The list also helps her to remember what she wants to discuss. She is getting forgetful these days, a sign of the menopause, she thinks.

2. She is seeing the doctor today because:

- she has had an intermittent dull pain (3/10) in her right calf, worse on standing up from gardening, since her sciatica 8 months ago. The pain does not interrupt sleep, but is an irritating niggle that rarely interferes with everyday activities. She wants to know if she should continue with the exercises the physiotherapist gave her, or whether she needs to see the physiotherapist again for further assessment and treatment.
- she still has an intermittent hoarse voice, but things are much better. Dr Brown spoke to her about reducing her alcohol intake and taking lansoprazole 30 mg for 1 month. This has helped but she has run out of tablets. A repeat script is required but she doesn't know if she should take 15 mg or 30 mg of lansoprazole now.
- she had blood tests done. Dr Brown wanted to check that she was not anaemic or diabetic or had thyroid problems, possible causes of her tiredness. She does not believe she has these conditions. Dr Brown wanted the other tests as 'a general health screen in the over 40's'. When told about the raised fasting glucose, she is adamant that she had fasted, and she is surprised and slightly worried by the result: what does it mean, and what does she need to do about it? She does not have symptoms of DM. No one in her family has DM.
- she is worried about her menopausal symptoms: feeling low, tired, no sex drive, weight gain and irregular periods for the last 4 months. Flushing occurs, but infrequently, so this is not a major issue. Mrs SW feels she lacks the energy to exercise, socialize, and make more friends. If she socialized more, she'd not drink at home during the evening. She wants to get her energy back.
- she attributes her lack of energy to the menopause – her 'idea'
- she is concerned about getting a DVT from HRT seeing that she already has a 'weak calf'

- she expects to be told about the pros and cons of HRT; she does not expect a prescription for HRT today, but she does expect a prescription for lansoprazole

3. Additional information:

- if the doctor offers her a prescription for HRT, she says she'd like to read up on it first. She'd also like to consider alternatives such as St John's Wort or valerian for sleep. She expects the doctor to signpost her to suitable information.

Approach to be taken

A. Data gathering, examination and clinical assessment skills

1. Define the clinical problem: clarify why the patient has presented today
The doctor:
- makes use of the existing patient information provided prior to the consultation
- empathises with Mrs SW's comments about needing to make a list because of her 'poor memory'
- asks the patient to read out the whole list to gauge which problems need urgent attention, which can be dealt with quickly, and which may need attention at a later date. One-way of dealing with the list may be to respond with *"Ok, that sounds like a reasonable list, all of which need attention. I also need to talk to you about your blood results. Shall we start with that and see how we get on in our ten minutes. If it's Ok with you, we'll also make a plan for dealing with those things we may not have time for today."*
- asks questions to explore how reliable the fasting blood glucose result is and makes arrangements for a glucose tolerance test (GTT)
- asks open questions to explore what Mrs SW means by menopausal symptoms, which symptoms have the greatest adverse impact on her life and what her expectations of treatment are, thereby eliciting the story of lacking energy and the expectation of treatment to restore her drive
- asks closed questions to clarify details about her periods, and possible contra-indications to HRT
- asks about red flags for calf pain (recent swelling or pain, recent long periods of immobility), and hoarse voice (particularly hoarseness that deteriorated over the past month despite proton pump inhibitors)
- discovers Mrs SW's idea that her lack of energy is due to the menopause, her concern about the risk of DVT with HRT, and her expectation for further information about HRT and a prescription for a lansoprazole

2. Performs an appropriate physical or mental examination
- In this case, an examination is not required.

B. Clinical management skills

3. Make an appropriate working diagnosis
The doctor, based on the history, makes a working diagnosis of:
- possible disorders of glucose metabolism requiring further investigation (GGT)
- peri-menopausal symptoms

4. *Explain the problem to the patient using appropriate language*
   The doctor:
   - explains that a diagnosis should not be made from a single blood test – the doctor organises a GTT, appropriately refers to the phlebotomist and gives clear instructions to the patient
   - provides information on the treatment of peri-menopausal symptoms: indicates that HRT may increase energy levels, SSRI's may help with flushing and valerian may help sleep; St John's wort is an enzyme inducer and may interfere with prescribed medication
   - explains the risks and benefits of HRT in appropriate language, and addresses the patient's particular concern regarding the risk of DVT on HRT
   - checks the patient's understanding at each point – if understanding is good, the doctor moves forward to the next item on the patient's list
   - prescribes an appropriate dose of lansoprazole for one month and negotiates review
   - negotiates review of the calf pain, explaining that a thorough reassessment of the sciatica and calf pain is required prior to making a decision regarding referral to physiotherapy. Alternatively, if the physiotherapy department had offered the patient an open-access appointment on discharge, she could call them directly for advice.

5. *Provide holistic care and use resources effectively*
   The doctor:
   - prioritises the issues effectively
   - makes balanced plans which are either doctor- or patient-centred as appropriate; for example, dealing with the raised fasting glucose is doctor-centred and dealing with the peri-menopausal symptoms is patient-centred
   - discusses conventional and complementary medicines, if Mrs SW is interested in the latter, for the treatment of her peri-menopausal symptoms; advice follows national or local guidelines (http://cks.library.nhs.uk/menopause)

6. *Prescribe appropriately*
   The doctor:
   - is aware of national and local guidelines (http://cks.library.nhs.uk/dyspepsia_proven_gord)
   - checks the patient's understanding of the medication and the amounts of medication required

7. *Specify the conditions and interval for follow-up*
   The doctor:
   - signposts Mrs SW to information on the menopause
   - offers a follow-up appointment to discuss issues not dealt with today; in particular, review of the voice hoarseness / GORD and calf pain / sciatica is arranged

C. Interpersonal skills: know and treat this patient

8. *Achieve rapport*
   The doctor:
   - listens attentively to Mrs SW's recitation of her list without interruption, acknowledging that concern for her ability to remember everything prompted its writing
   - understands her request for information on HRT, a repeat script for a PPI and review of her sciatica; the doctor is sympathetic and outlines his intention to address these issues today and at future appointments
   - displays empathy to her lack of energy and supports her in her attempt to change her lifestyle
   - is non-judgemental about the patient's alcohol intake and congratulates her on the reduction she's made
   - addresses the patient's specific concerns and expectations

9. *Give the patient the opportunity to be involved in significant management decisions*
   The doctor:
   - encourages autonomy and opinions – provides Mrs SW with a brief outline on treatment options and signposts to appropriate resources on HRT management
   - suggests further appointments with appropriate members of the PCT for future review

Debrief

Discuss how the doctor could, if needed, improve his performance. In particular, assess whether the doctor:

- negotiated the patient's list? Was this done in a sensitive manner?
- established and maintained rapport? If so, how?
- addressed Mrs SW's specific expectations? If so, how?
- discussed and signposted to appropriate HRT, including CAM?
- safety netted? If so, how?

If the consultation over-ran, did the doctor:

- spend too much time negotiating the list?
- ask too many questions about all the presenting issues before deciding on the ones to tackle?
- provide detailed information when outlining the main points would have sufficed? Remember that if the actor–patient is unhappy with the amount and detail of information provided, they are briefed to press the issue. In this case, the actor-patient would have been briefed to leave the appointment with a script for her PPI, a follow-up blood test, some information on treatments for the menopause and a strategy for tackling her on-going calf pain/sciatica. An acceptable strategy would be *"let's discuss this further at a follow-up appointment, which you can arrange, at your convenience, with the receptionist."*

Revising data gathering

What questions could the doctor ask to discover the patient's ideas, and expectations? How could the doctor address the patient's concerns and health beliefs?

- Ideas: *"You mention making a list to help you remember? What do you think is making you forgetful? Do you think that feeling low and lacking energy is due to the menopause?"*
- Concerns: *"Your calf pain sounds like on-going sciatica – nerve pain, rather than a DVT. HRT affects the blood and slightly increases the risk of clotting in the veins. HRT should not make your nerve pain worse and your sciatica does not increase your risk of clotting."*
- Expectations: *"Your list allows us to prioritise things so we can tackle them logically. If we can't get through everything, please remind me that I definitely have to discuss your blood results; what do you definitely have to leave with today?"*
- Health beliefs: *"I agree that your symptoms sound like the menopause. How we treat the menopause depends on which symptoms are troubling you most. HRT is probably better for the lack of energy and irregular bleeding, but low mood and hot flushes could be treated with Prozac-type medication, while poor sleep could be treated with regular exercise or valerian. Let me briefly outline each option for you and then give you some written information. How does that sound?"*

Test your theoretical knowledge

For each of the following statements, answer true (T) or false (F).

Regarding hoarseness:
1. Hoarseness due to upper respiratory tract infections resolves spontaneously
2. Hoarseness due to hypothyroidism is likely to resolve with thyroxine treatment
3. Paralysis of the recurrent laryngeal nerve, due to surgical trauma or malignancy, presents with hoarseness
4. If hoarseness persists for more than 6 weeks, refer to a chest physician to exclude oropharyngeal malignancy
5. The effect of inhaled steroids on hoarseness is not dose-related

Relevant literature

www.patient.co.uk/showdoc/40000966/

http://cks.library.nhs.uk/menopause

http://cks.library.nhs.uk/dyspepsia_proven_gord

Case 20 - Dyspepsia

Brief to the doctor

Mr ST, a 45 year old man, has seen you twice in the past 3 months for dyspepsia. One month ago you gave him a prescription for omeprazole 20 mg once daily for 28 days.

Patient summary

Name	ST
Date of birth (Age)	45
Social and family history	Married
Past medical history	3 months ago: GP consultation: "*4months' dyspepsia. No red flags. Smokes 15/day. Alc – 18 units/week. Intermittent diclofenac for back. OTC Gaviscon helps. OE - NAD. Advised – lose weight, stop smoking, no late meals. Stop diclofenac. Gaviscon prn 500mls.*"
	1 month ago: GP consultation: "*Above not helped. Had partic bad episode and OTC ranitidine helped. Back is OK with paracetamol. Still smoking. Has lost some wt – congratulated. Abdo soft. No red flags, so 1m trial PPI. Omeprazole 20mg od x28. Rev 1m*"
Current medication	Omeprazole 20 mg od Diclofenac 50 mg 1 tds prn for back pain
Investigations	3months ago:
BMI	29.3
BP	134/86
Tobacco	15/day
Alcohol	18 units/wk

Tasks for the doctor

In this case, the tasks are to:
1. ascertain Mr ST's response to the PPI trial
2. agree a management plan including lifestyle changes

Brief to the patient – more about the patient

1. Profile:

- Mr ST is 45 years old. He works in the planning department at the local council. He married with 3 teenage children
- His father died 10 years ago of an MI aged 60; mother alive, hypertensive
- Smokes 15/day – he has tried patches and gum in the past, but was never cigarette free for more than 3 weeks
- drinks 18 units/week (wine)

2. He is seeing the doctor today because:

- he has had indigestion for 7 months – the response to omeprazole has been 'miraculous'
- he would like to continue taking the tablets

3. Additional information:

- If the doctor asks specifically:
  - his indigestion symptoms are: upper abdominal pain between meals with some belching. The pain has woken him at night a couple of times in the past. Symptoms worse after big or late meals. No nausea, vomiting, haematemesis, heartburn, dysphagia.
  - he has lost a few pounds
  - he still gets intermittent back pain, but since being told to stop taking diclofenac, he has been able to control this reasonably well with paracetamol and exercises. He thinks this has been a good move, because it has made him do his exercises and watch his posture rather than 'just take a tablet and mask the pain'.
  - he is not concerned he has anything other than plain indigestion and he does not want any investigations
  - he has heard about *H. pylori* and wonders whether he should be tested as this might give him life-long cure
- He enjoys smoking and finds it helps him relax. If the doctor can present him with evidence that he has other risk factors for heart disease, he might be persuaded to give stopping another try.
- He could easily be persuaded to lose weight and change his diet.
- He would like to be more physically active and is open to suggestions on how to lead a more physically active life. He drives to work, dropping the children off at school on the way. They live on the edge of town, just too far to walk into town easily.

Approach to be taken

A. Data gathering, examination and clinical assessment skills

1. Define the clinical problem: clarify why the patient has presented today
The doctor:
- reads the patient information provided prior to the consultation
- asks open questions to explore how Mr ST responded to the omeprazole and whether he believes the lifestyle changes he made previously helped: *"How have things been since I saw you last?"*
- asks closed questions to exclude red flag symptoms signalling the need for referral
- discovers Mr ST's desire to keep taking omeprazole: *"Have you any ideas about what we should do now?"*
- clarifies whether Mr ST would like further tests: *"Have you heard about any investigations or tests for this?"*

2. Performs an appropriate physical or mental examination
- In this case, an examination is not required.

B. Clinical management skills

3. Make an appropriate working diagnosis
- The doctor, based on the history, makes a working diagnosis of uninvestigated dyspepsia with no red flags; Mr ST tells you that he is happy with this diagnosis.

4. Explain the problem to the patient using appropriate language
The doctor:
- having quickly established Mr ST's response to omeprazole, addresses his agenda: wanting to keep taking omeprazole
- provides some information on the effectiveness of lifestyle changes in the management of dyspepsia

5. Provide holistic care and use resources effectively
The doctor:
- informs Mr ST about *H. pylori* testing, eradication treatment and success rates and ascertains whether he would like to explore this treatment option
- discusses the pros and cons of using omeprazole long-term, either continuously or intermittently
- explores Mr ST's ideas about smoking and the benefits of stopping smoking: *"Have you any thoughts about how smoking might be affecting you?"*
- identifies other risk factors for CVD: FH, overweight, relative lack of exercise and uses this to try to motivate Mr ST to stop smoking, lose weight and lead a more physically active lifestyle

- congratulates Mr ST for managing his back pain without diclofenac – this is an opportunity to reinforce a message that self-management can be very effective

6. *Prescribe appropriately*
The doctor:

- is aware of national and local guidelines – NICE (2004, revised 2005) *Dyspepsia: management of dyspepsia in adults in primary care*
- negotiates an appropriate treatment option:
  - ○ return to self-management (as per NICE guidelines)
  - ○ intermittent PPI use
  - ○ *H. pylori* testing
- offers smoking cessation advice
- offers advice on diet, weight loss and increased physical activity

7. *Specify the conditions and interval for follow-up*
The doctor:

- signposts Mr ST to information on CVD risk factors
- offers a follow-up appointment either with a doctor or with a nurse to discuss smoking cessation and other lifestyle modifications
- arranges a follow up appointment to review the *H. pylori* test result
- safety nets – informs Mr ST about dyspepsia 'red-flag' symptoms
- confirms understanding – *"Do you have any questions?"*

C. Interpersonal skills: know and treat this patient

8. *Achieve rapport*
The doctor:

- listens actively and explores the patient's health ideas, concerns and expectations
- in particular, explores and clarifies Mr ST's beliefs about medication, smoking and motivation for stopping smoking
- explores ways to motivate the patient to lose weight and to become more physically active
- displays empathy and is non-judgemental about Mr ST's weight and smoking

9. *Give the patient the opportunity to be involved in significant management decisions*
The doctor:

- actively confirms the patient's understanding of the dyspepsia and CVD risk factors: *"Does all this make sense to you?"*
- shares thoughts and involves patient in deciding which management option to select
- encourages autonomy and opinions – provides him with information so he feels able to understand self-management for himself and his family
- supports and congratulates his self-management of his back pain

Debrief

Discuss how the doctor could, if needed, improve his performance. In particular, assess how the doctor:

- negotiated an appropriate management plan for dyspepsia
- discussed CVD risk factors
- tried to motivate Mr ST to stop smoking
- structured the consultation and used the time appropriately

Revising data gathering

What questions could the doctor ask to discover the patient's ideas, concerns, expectations and health beliefs?

- Ideas: "*I understand that you are keen to continue on omeprazole; have you thought about other ways to treat your symptoms?*"
- Concerns: "*You don't seem keen on stopping smoking. Are there any particular reasons?*"
- Expectations: "*It seems that you are not very happy with your current diet; would you like to discuss how it could be improved?*"
- Health beliefs: "*You know that smoking increases your risk of heart disease, but there are other factors as well. Would you like to check over these and see if any apply to you?*"

Test your theoretical knowledge

For each of the following statements, answer true (T) or false (F).

1. A minimum 4 week wash-out period following PPI use is required before testing for *H. pylori* with a breath test
2. Patients over 55 whose symptoms persist despite *H. pylori* eradication or acid suppression treatment should be considered for endoscopy
3. Cognitive behaviour therapy may reduce dyspepsia symptoms in the short-term
4. For patients with persistent symptoms, but no red-flag symptoms, testing for and treating *H. pylori* is more cost effective than further management based on endoscopy
5. The prevalence of *H. pylori* in the UK is around 40%

Relevant literature

Delaney BC, Qume M, Moayyedi P, *et al.* (2008) *Helicobacter pylori* test and treat versus proton pump inhibitor in initial management of dyspepsia in primary care: multicentre randomised controlled trial (MRC-CUBE trial). *BMJ,* **336:** 651–654.

NICE (2004, revised 2005) *Dyspepsia: management of dyspepsia in adults in primary care* (CG17): www.nice.org.uk/Guidance/CG17).

Preparing for the nMRCGP Clinical Skills Assessment (CSA)

In this section, we shall discuss:
- how to use the mock cases
- information about the CSA, including:
  o the structure of the CSA
  o what happens on the exam day
  o the marking of the CSA
  o preparing for the CSA

How to use the mock cases

The mock cases in this section of the book are intended to help candidates who are working together in a group to prepare for the CSA.
- The candidate / 'doctor' only has access to the pages containing the patient summary and tasks for the doctor.
- The 'patient' has access to the pages containing *Brief to the patient – more about the patient*.
- After running the case, the candidates should analyse their performance by answering the questions contained in the *Debrief* section. This should highlight what was done well and which aspects of the consultation the doctor needs to improve prior to the CSA.
- The consultation runs smoothly if the doctor has sufficient theoretical knowledge to apply to the case to move the consultation forward. Hence, each mock case ends with a *Test your theoretical knowledge* section to identify learning needs.

Information about the CSA

The structure of CSA
The CSA is one of the three components of the nMRCGP assessment. It is designed to test a doctor's ability to ***integrate*** and ***apply*** clinical, professional, communication and practical skills appropriate for general practice, "to produce a consultation that is meaningful to both patient and doctor and which moves the patient forward towards a justifiable management of their presenting problem" (Hawthorne, 2007).

What happens on exam day
- On the day of the examination, at the examination venue, each candidate is given a consulting room.
- The candidate is briefed to treat the examination session as if he is a locum doctor.
- He is to interact with the patient and not the examiner, who will remain a silent observer.

- The candidate's surgery has thirteen booked patients who enter his consulting room when the buzzer sounds.
- At the end of 10 minutes, the buzzer sounds to signal the departure of the patient.
- There is a two minute gap between consultations.
- Twelve patients are true examination cases on which the candidate is assessed. One is a 'trial station' in which new clinical scenarios are trailed. The candidiate will not know which is the trial case.
- There will be a short break in the middle of surgery.

The marking of CSA

The patients, played by trained actors, will move from room to room, together with the examiner for that case. Each examiner will mark the same case all day, thus providing standardised marking.

Each case is marked in three domains, all have equal weighting.
- *Data gathering, examination and clinical assessment skills*: the ability to take a targeted history and perform a focussed physical examination. Candidates are expected to be knowledgeable and skillful in their examination techniques and in the appropriate use of medical instruments. Marks are awarded for the fluency with which procedures are performed.
- *Clinical management skills*: in line with current accepted British general practice.
- *Interpersonal skills:* the candidate shows an ability to engage patients in the consultation, using recognised interpersonal skills, such as enquiring about the patient's health beliefs and incorporating these into the explanation given to the patient. Some cases also assess the candidate's ability to value patients' contributions, and to respect their autonomy and decision-making.

The pass mark is set as the standard required to practise independently as a licensed GP. The candidate is then given an overall grade, namely a Clear Pass, Marginal Pass, Marginal Fail or Clear Fail.

In very simple terms, data-gathering is about **how** you get to the 'nub' of the presenting problem; clinical management is about **what** you do to move the problem forward; and interpersonal skills is about **how** you go about doing it.

Each case is written to focus on a particular 'nub'. The marking schedule, using positive and negative indicators of practice, reflects this nub. Please refer to video cases 8 to 13 for examples of the marking schedule.

Preparing for CSA

Do the job. The CSA cases are all written by GPs active in the UK National Health Service and reflect real-life presentations. Therefore, candidates with some experience in NHS general practice should not have difficulty with the exam. The RCGP recommends that candidates first complete at least 6 months of UK NHS GP practice before sitting the exam.

Read the website. Candidates are advised to read the Curriculum Statements from the RCGP website. Each curriculum statement has a section on common and important conditions and cases are quite likely to be based on one of these.

Analyse your consultations. Candidates are advised to video their own consultations, watch them with a colleague, and analyse them for the clinical approach and interpersonal skills displayed. Alternatively, candidates may work in small groups, practising mock cases, such as the ones contained in this section of the book.

Practise clinical examinations. Candidates are advised to practise the focussed examinations that are most likely to be tested, such as assessment of a limb, chest or abdomen. Some examinations, such as intimate examinations on a role player, or examinations that might cause discomfort if repeated are less likely to be tested. Candidates are advised to be familiar and confident with medical equipment, such as otoscopes.

Interpret data. Candidates are advised to become familiar with the letters GPs receive from secondary care, and test results such as ECGs, spirometry, blood tests, urinalysis, skin scrapings, and swabs. Candidates need to ensure that they can interpret results correctly and explain them to a patient.

The mock CSA cases in this section of the book includes cases that require candidates to practise physical examination and interpret test results.

Additional reading

Malik S (2006) An OSCE actress. *BMJ Career Focus*, **332**: 110.

Ms Malik describes her experience as an OCSE actress, how she was briefed to play the case, and what examiners asked of her regarding the candidates. She also gives her tips on how candidates should prepare:

> "I would suggest that if you can sense the acting patient is not happy with the situation then you should ask: *"Is there anything I've said that is confusing or not clear or that you want explained again?"* Another tip is to have a mental checklist of questions prepared and if you find yourself in an awkward situation, go back to where you left off in the list."

Relevant literature

Hawthorne K (2007) Introduction to the cases in the Clinical Skills Assessment. RCGP website: www.rcgp-curriculum.org.uk/nmrgcp/csa/csa_cases.aspx

Simpson RG (2007) Preparing for practice: nMRCGP and the Clinical Skills Assessment. *Update,* **75**: 36–37.

Royal College of General Practitioners nMRCGP website:
www.rcgp-curriculum.org.uk/examinations_and_assessment.aspx, particularly:

- www.rcgp-curriculum.org.uk/PDF/curr_1_Curriculum_Statement_Being_a_GP.pdf
  for the GP curriculum – the core statement
- www.rcgp.org.uk/pdf/curriculum_Guide_for_Learners_and_Teachers.pdf for in-
  depth reading of learning outcomes for general practice

Mock case 1 – Menopausal symptoms

Brief to the doctor

Mrs KC is a 46 year old woman who had blood tests done three weeks ago. She returns to discuss the results and possible treatment options.

Patient summary

Name	KC
Date of birth (Age)	46
Social and Family History	Has two teenage daughters from her 1st marriage and one son (9 years) from her 2nd marriage Works as an assistant in a hospice
Past medical history	Endometrial ablation (6 months ago) Menorrhagia (2 years ago) Post-natal depression (9 years ago)
Past medication	Zoladex implant 3.6 mg (6 months ago)

Consultation note by Dr Brown (4 weeks ago):
'Menopausal symptoms: hot flushes, feeling irritable, vaginal dryness, reduced energy and reduced sleep, waking early and ruminating. Has a stressful job at hospice. Finding it difficult not having periods after ablation. O/E: anxious lady with some pressure of speech. Near to tears at one point. Plan: for FSH, LH, progestogen and cholesterol bloods. ?menopause ?low mood worsening symptoms.'

Blood tests	Tests were done 2 weeks ago
Fasting glucose	6.2 (3–5.5)
Total cholesterol	6.5 mmol/l
HDL	1.2
Plasma oestradiol	42 pmol/l (40–1930)
Serum progestogen	1 mmol/l (14–90)
Plasma prolactin	77 mU/l (60–620)
Plasma FSH	42 IU/l (1.5–33)
Plasma LH	32.5 IU/l) (2–10)
	Test done 2 years ago
TSH	3.64 mU/l (0.35 – 5.5)

Tasks for the doctor

In this case, the tasks are to:

- summarise the presenting problems: first, an isolated raised fasting glucose, and secondly, symptoms and tests suggesting the menopause
- provide sufficient information to move the consultation forward
- involve the patient in the management plan

Brief to the patient – more about the patient

1. Profile:

- Mrs KC is a 46 year old woman who started work at the local hospice a year ago
- she started nursing studies, as a mature student, but found juggling home and studies too difficult, so she discontinued the studies and took up a nursing assistant post at the hospice
- she is married to a younger man, aged 37, and they have a good relationship
- her 2nd teenage daughter left home recently to start university and she feels lonely without her daughters

2. She is seeing the doctor today because:

- she wants to know the results of her recent blood tests – she is adamant that she fasted for the test
- she does not want to believe she is peri-menopausal (*"that's getting old, isn't it?"*) and hopes to put symptoms down to 'stress'
- several issues cause 'stress': feeling lonely at home, doing 'menial', boring, repetitive housework, and dealing with dying people at work
- her husband is busy working towards a promotion; she has spoken to him but feels that he has *"not listened"*
- she has not had regular periods, only occasional light bleeds since her endometrial ablation and this makes her feel *"even less of a woman"*
- her main symptoms are fragility of mood and mood swings; *"little things like leaving the toothpaste uncapped"* upset her
- hot flushes occur perhaps once or twice per week and she feels she can cope with them; however, she is tired, despite 8 hours of sleep, and would like to have more energy

3. Additional information:

- if the doctor discusses HRT with her, she would like to know the pros and cons of HRT. She does not have contra-indications to HRT, but wonders if she is at increased risk of breast cancer if her aunt (her mother's sister) had breast cancer at age 52.
- if SSRIs are discussed, she wants to know if the doctor thinks *"it is all in the head?"*
- Mrs KC has come across alternative medications at the hospice and is particularly keen on 'natural remedies'. She would like more information on natural treatments for the menopause and she asks for your opinion on phyto-oestrogens.

Debrief

Discuss how the doctor could, if needed, improve his performance. In particular, assess whether the doctor:

- established rapport? If so, how?
- addressed Mrs KC's specific concerns about breast cancer and being perceived as a 'headcase'? If so, how?
- addressed Mrs KC's expectations for information on natural remedies for the menopause?
- discussed the evidence base for HRT and natural remedies using simple and jargon free language?
- involved the patient in the management plan?

If the consultation over-ran, did the doctor:

- repeat certain questions when taking the history?
- provide very detailed explanations?
- address issues the patient was not concerned about?

Test your theoretical knowledge

For each of the following statements, answer true (T) or false (F).

Regarding menopause and mood disorders

1. Although most women transition to menopause without experiencing psychiatric problems, an estimated 20% have depression at some point during menopause
2. Insomnia occurs in 40–50% of women during the peri-menopause
3. Hot flushes are often blamed for patients' sleep problems; however, results of polysomnographic studies have disproved this theory
4. Postmenopausal women experience a decline in melatonin and an increase in growth hormone levels; the former affects sleep
5. A second peak in the incidence of schizophrenia is noted among women aged 45–50 years; this second peak is not observed in men
6. An FSH level >25 IU/l is often used as a marker of menopausal changes
7. Paroxetine, venlafaxine, clonidine and gabapentin have been shown to reduce hot flushes

Relevant literature

www.emedicine.com/med/TOPIC3756.HTM

Mock case 2 – Schoolgirl with hay fever

Brief to the doctor

AL's mother consults you to ask for a letter for her daughter's school confirming that AL suffers from hay fever and that this may affect her performance in her GCSE exams. AL is 15 years old. When your receptionist advised AL's mother that there might be a charge for a letter she was not very happy.

Patient summary

Name	AL
Date of birth (Age)	15
Social and Family History	Student Lives with her parents and younger brother aged 11
Past medical history	Hay fever since age 4 Recurrent tonsillitis age 7–10 years
Current medication	Cetirizine tablet 10 mg once daily

Tasks for the doctor

In this case, the tasks are to:
- confirm AL's diagnosis and assess how well her symptoms are controlled and hence the likelihood of them affecting her exam performance
- consider changing the management of AL's hay fever
- provide a letter for AL's school, and explain the reason for a charge for this to AL's mother

Brief to the patient – more about the patient

1. Profile:

- AL's mother is 45, she is a department manager in a department store in the town
- she has two children – a girl AL aged 15 and a boy TL aged 11
- AL has suffered from hay fever since the age of 4 and this has always been managed by oral antihistamines. For the past few years, AL's symptoms have been reasonably well controlled on this medication, but on occasions in the past couple of years, her mother has bought her OTC eye drops and a nose spray from the local chemist to supplement the antihistamines.
- AL's symptoms are a blocked, runny nose with frequent sneezing, itchy sore eyes, tickly roof of her mouth and disturbed sleep due to discomfort and blocked nose; she does not have any cough or wheezing
- AL experiences no side effects from the antihistamines
- AL will be taking GCSEs in 2 months' time and her teacher has advised her mother to get a letter from the doctor confirming that AL gets bad hay fever and asking that this should be taken into account when assessing her performance in the exams

2. AL's mother is seeing the doctor today because:

- she would like the doctor to provide a letter for the school free of charge

3. Additional information:

- If the doctor asks specifically:
  - there is no family history of atopy
  - the receptionist has advised her that there is a charge for the letter, but she believes that this is not fair as AL is a child and entitled to free prescriptions, health care, education and even dentistry! AL's mother will ask the doctor what s/he would do if the parents could not afford to pay for the letter as this would potentially disadvantage a child from an apparent poor background, which she considers is surely unfair.
  - she does not feel AL's hay fever is controlled optimally, but AL does not like using nose sprays and is not keen on self-administering eye drops (the school will not administer medication to pupils)

Debrief

This case tests the doctor's ability to:
- deal with a proxy consultation
- manage a patient's anger
- negotiate an agreed management plan

Discuss how the doctor could, if needed, improve his performance. In particular, assess whether the doctor:
- structured the consultation
- used the available time appropriately
- obtained the mother's agreement on managing AL's symptoms
- dealt with the mother's feelings about being charged for a letter

Test your theoretical knowledge

For each of the following statements, answer true (T) or false (F).

1. Food allergens do not tend to cause allergic rhinoconjunctivitis symptoms
2. In most cases of chronic rhinoconjunctivitis no allergen can be identified
3. There is no evidence to support the belief that allergic rhinoconjunctivitis in children can cause learning difficulties
4. The commonest local side effect of intranasal glucocorticosteroid sprays is epistaxis
5. Symptoms of rhinitis may be induced by drugs such as oral contraceptives and aspirin

Relevant literature

British Society for Allergy and Clinical Immunology ENT Sub-Committee (2000) *Rhinitis Management Guidelines,* 3rd Edition. London.

De Groot H, Brand PLP, Fokkens WF, Berger MY. (2007) Allergic rhinoconjunctivitis in children. *BMJ,* **335:** 985–988.

Mock case 3 – Oligomenorrhoea

Brief to the doctor

Miss PA is a 28 year old woman who was advised to see a doctor by the practice nurse.

Patient summary

Name	PA
Date of birth (Age)	28
Social and Family History	Works as an administrative assistant at a local timber merchants Plays rugby for the local amateur team
Past medical history	Thoracic back pain 3 months ago Ankle pain 9 months ago
Past medication	Diclofenac 50 mg thrice daily (9 months ago) Omeprazole 20 mg once daily (9 months ago)

Consultation note by practice nurse (last week):
'LMP 12 of last month. No previous smear abnormalities. Very irregular menstrual cycle. 4–5 months between periods. Not currently sexually active. Never smoked tobacco.
O/E: medium speculum. Transition zone seen. Smear taken. Nullip – bled slightly on contact. BP 132/80.
Plan: will write to patient with smear results. Advised to see GP to discuss periods.'

Tasks for the doctor

In this case, the tasks are to:
- understand the process by which Miss PA decided to consult and how this could affect the consultation outcome
- negotiate a shared understanding of the problem and its management with the patient, so that she is empowered to look after her own health
- demonstrate commitment to health promotion, while recognising the potential tension between this role and the patient's own agenda

Brief to the patient – more about the patient

1. Profile:

- Miss PA is a 28 year old woman who works as an administrative assistant at the local timber merchants
- she has not been in a relationship for 3 years
- she plays rugby and runs to keep fit; despite her exercise and attendance at a weekly slimming club, she has found it difficult to lose the 12 kg she gained 3 years ago, after her last relationship ended
- she says her family members are healthy, but if polycystic ovarian syndrome (PCOS) is mentioned, she says her sister (age 45) may have this

2. She is seeing the doctor today because:

- she was advised by the nurse that it is not a good idea to have only three periods in a year, but she is not sure why this is a problem
- she stopped taking the combined pill (Pill) three years ago. For the first 2 years, her periods occurred every 2 months. In the last year, she has had a period every 4 months. Bleeding is light and unpredictable. She is not troubled by the irregular bleeding and, until the nurse mentioned it, had not perceived a problem.
- when questioned, she admits to hair growing on her chest and the anterior aspect of her neck
- she has an oily T-zone but no acne
- she does not have symptoms of diabetes
- she is not in a relationship and fertility is not an issue
- her main symptoms are scant, infrequent periods, difficulty losing weight and hirsutism
- she is not troubled by these symptoms. However, she is slightly concerned by the nurse's reaction – does she have a gynaecological problem? Are tests needed? What can she do to improve her health?

3. Additional information:

- she admits to knowing very little about PCOS when questioned, but she is keen to know more and requests information
- if tests are requested, she wants to know what the results could mean; she asks if these will affect her insurance medical as she plans to buy a house soon
- if weight loss is mentioned, she says it has been a struggle to keep the weight off over the last 3 years and she is not hopeful about losing more weight

Debrief

Discuss how the doctor could, if needed, improve his performance. In particular, assess whether the doctor:

- communicated well, that is, did he establish rapport, address the patient's expectations, use jargon-free language and involve the patient in the management plan
- formulated an appropriate diagnosis and ruled out serious illness
- obtained consent for on-going investigation, that is, was the doctor able to share information about the condition and insurance premiums in an honest and unbiased manner?
- demonstrated respect for the practice nurse's role in highlighting the potential health problem

If the consultation ran to time, did the doctor:
- take a systematic and sufficiently detailed history?
- provide an explanation defining a safe number of minimum bleeds per year and long term health screening?
- address the concern about insurance premiums in an empathetic manner?

Test your theoretical knowledge

For each of the following statements, answer true (T) or false (F).

Regarding PCOS
1. PCOS is often complicated by chronic anovulatory infertility and hyperandrogenism with the clinical manifestation of oligomenorrhoea, hirsutism and acne
2. Women with this condition have the same prevalence of sleep apnoea when compared to the general population
3. A raised luteinising hormone/follicle-stimulating hormone ratio and biochemical signs of hyperandrogenism are two of the three criteria diagnostic of PCOS
4. The recommended baseline screening tests are thyroid function tests, a serum prolactin and a free androgen index
5. Because oligo- or amenorrhoea in women with PCOS may predispose to endometrial hyperplasia and later carcinoma; treatment with progestogens to induce a withdrawal bleed at least every 3–4 months is recommended
6. Orlistat and sibutramine have not been shown to significantly reduce hyperandrogenism in women with PCOS
7. A glucose tolerance test (GTT) is advised in women with a body mass index greater than 30 if fertility is an issue

Relevant literature

www.emedicine.com/med/TOPIC3756.HTM

Mock case 4 – Metastatic prostate cancer

Brief to the doctor

Mr CN is an 83 year old man who has been a life-long patient of the practice. He and his wife have sent a bottle of whisky to the practice every Christmas for as long as anyone can remember.

He was diagnosed with cancer of the prostate 5 years ago and treated with external beam radiotherapy. One year ago he relapsed with local symptoms and spinal pain and was started on hormonal treatment. However, his cancer has proved refractory to this treatment and he has recently been fully assessed by the specialist multidisciplinary team and offered chemotherapy. He is coming to see you, with his wife, to talk about his recent outpatient appointment.

Patient summary

Name	CN
Date of birth (Age)	83 years
Social and Family History	Married to MN, aged 81
Past medical history	Age 71 years – Left TKR Age 74 years – Right THR Age 78 years – Cancer of prostate. Radical radiotherapy
	1 year ago – Back pain, urinary symptoms, PSA rising. Bony (L spine) and intrapelvic metastases confirmed on MRI. Started gonaderelin analogue therapy.
	6 weeks ago – Seen in outpatients: "*He does not seem to be responding to hormonal treatment any more – his local symptoms and bone pain are now progressing and his general condition is deteriorating. His wife now needs to assist him to get about. We will repeat his MRI to assess tumour bulk and review.*"
	1 week ago – Seen in outpatients: "*Repeat MRI shows progression of pelvic and bone (L spine and Rt ilium) metastases. He has hormone refractory disease and has been offered chemotherapy to slow progression of disease*

and hopefully relieve some local symptoms. He has gone away to discuss this with his wife and family. We have arranged to see him again in 2 weeks."

Current medication   Co-codamol 30/500 2 tablets qds
Lactulose 10–15 mls bd

Investigations   None

Tasks for the doctor

In this case, the tasks are to:
- review Mr CN's current symptoms and medication
- explore his feelings about future treatment
- offer support to Mr CN and his family

Brief to the patient – more about the patient

1. Profile:

- Mr CN is an 83 year old man, married to MN, who is fit and well
- when seen in outpatients 6 weeks ago he was told that his cancer was not responding to treatment and he needed further tests. Last week he was told his cancer had spread and was offered chemotherapy to slow down the progression of his disease, but was told that this was not to be considered curative.
- His current symptoms are:
    - he feels tired and is losing weight
    - he has become increasingly frail and can no longer go out alone
    - he has hesitancy and dribbling stream and is sometimes incontinent of urine. He finds the latter particularly distressing and demeaning. He gets up 4 or 5 times every night to pass water.
    - he has constant back and right hip pain – the pain disturbs his sleep and he has taken to sleeping in the spare room so as not to disturb his wife, which they both find distressing

2. He is seeing the doctor today because:

- he does not want to have any further treatment. He feels that all the treatments offered to him will not improve the quality of his life. He has discussed this with his wife, and she respects his feelings and is supportive. His family have said that it his decision and they will support him whatever he decides.
- he would like to ask if he can refuse treatment and whether this will lead to a loss of follow-up support from the cancer and incontinence teams
- he would also like to know how he will be managed by the practice – medication, home visits, nursing and social service support

3. Additional information:

- If the doctor asks specifically:
    - he would like stronger painkillers, but is frightened that they will sedate him so that he cannot enjoy his final days
    - he is frightened of his pain being uncontrollable and his family having to witness him dying in extreme pain
    - he wants to die a dignified death at home and wants to know what services and support are available to enable this
- His wife is a quiet lady and takes no part in the consultation other than to confirm her husband's comments.
- He wants to thank the doctor and the practice for the support they have given him and his wife all their lives and asks if a representative of the practice, preferably his GP, would attend his funeral.

Debrief

This case tests the doctor's ability to:

- discuss death and terminal care with a patient and his wife in an open and supportive manner, exploring and addressing the patient's and his family's specific concerns and fears
- support a patient who has made a very difficult decision
- involve the appropriate elements of the PCT in the patient's care
- handle a difficult question about attending a patient's funeral
- prescribe appropriate analgesia

Discuss how the doctor could, if needed, improve his performance. In particular, assess whether the doctor:

- structured the consultation in order to use the available time appropriately
- established the patient's decision about refusing further treatment
- clarified the patient's fears about how the medical team will respond to his decision – "*What do you think the hospital will make of your choice?*"
- clarified the patient's wishes about future care – "*Have you any thoughts or concerns about what we can do to help you in the future?*"
- answered the patient's anxieties and concerns appropriately
- explored the patient's and his wife's fears, beliefs, ideas, concerns and expectations about support they would receive
- used appropriate language
- established empathy and support
- prescribed appropriate analgesia
- checked that the patient's concerns had been answered – "*Is there anything else we haven't covered?*"
- outlined the range of skills available in the PCT
- safety-netted by explaining when to take top-up analgesia, and how and when to access services during and outside normal working hours

Test your theoretical knowledge

For each of the following statements, answer true (T) or false (F).

1. Most patients with cancer cannot have their pain controlled effectively
2. Most patients commencing opioids in terminal care experience nausea and vomiting
3. Patients starting opioids for moderate to severe pain should be prescribed both softening and stimulant laxatives
4. Hypercalcaemia can mimic opioid side effects
5. NSAIDs should not be used due to their gastric side effects

Relevant literature

National Council for Palliative Care (2003) Guidance for managing cancer pain in adults.

Arroll B. (2007) Should doctors go to patients' funerals? *BMJ,* **334:** 1332.

Chochinov H. (2007) Dignity and the essence of medicine: the A, B, C, and D of dignity conserving care. *BMJ,* **334:** 184–187.

Mock case 5 – Period problems

Brief to the doctor

Mrs EH is a 30 year old Muslim woman who rarely consults. She is booked at the end of your surgery as a telephone consultation. The receptionist says the patient is concerned about a problem but, as she works full time, wondered if she could speak to you for advice.

Patient summary

Name	EH
Date of birth (Age)	30
Social and Family History	Married, no children Personal assistant to an executive
Past medical history	Discoid eczema
Past medication	Hydrocortisone 2% (8 months ago)

Consultation note by practice nurse (7 months ago):
'Routine smear taken. No previous abnormal smears. No hormonal contraceptives. Never smoked tobacco.
O/E: medium-long speculum. Transition zone seen. BMI 29.5. BP 125/71.
Plan: will write to patient with smear results. Pre-conception advice: no Pill x 3 months and is taking folic acid.'

Tasks for the doctor

In this case, the tasks are to:
- demonstrate a reasoned approach to the diagnosis of women's symptoms in a manner that is comfortable for both the patient and the GP
- use history to decide if further examination, incremental investigations and referral are needed
- demonstrate an understanding of the importance of risk factors in the diagnosis and management of women's problems
- be sensitive to the impact of culture and ethnicity on the perceived role of women in society and their attendant health beliefs, and tailor health care accordingly

Brief to the patient – more about the patient

1. Profile:

- Mrs EH is a 30 year old woman who works as personal assistant to an executive in the City of London, a job she enjoys
- she has been happily married for 4 years
- she eats healthily and keeps fit; she walks to and from the Docklands ferry each day (30 minutes each way)
- she says her father (age 57) and his two older sisters are diabetic, but mother and two siblings are all fine

2. She is calling the doctor today because:

- she has missed her last two periods but over-the-counter pregnancy tests done 1 week after each missed period were negative
- she usually has regular periods and bleeds for 4–5 days every 30 days
- she is due her next period in 2 weeks, while she is on holiday
- she stopped taking the combined pill (Pill) 20 months ago; within 2 months her cycle returned to 4/30; 10 months ago, she stopped using condoms and is trying to conceive
- she does not have symptoms of diabetes, has not lost or gained weight, and has not exercised excessively. She is not experiencing any undue stress. There are no symptoms to suggest thyroid disease, prolactin problems, auto-immune or gynaecological disease. There is no history of previous surgery or significant illness.
- she is slightly concerned about her difficulty in conceiving but thinks that with time, conception will occur
- her main symptom is the two missed periods with negative pregnancy tests – why is she missing periods?
- she is slightly concerned about getting a period while on holiday and hopes it arrives within the week, before she leaves. She wants to know if she has a gynaecological problem? Are tests needed? Are medicines needed?

3. Additional information:

- she is philosophical about her difficulties conceiving; this is not why she consults today
- if she is asked to come in for an examination, she talks about her long working hours and asks about surgery opening hours – does she really need to be examined? If she speaks to a male doctor, she asks if she could make the appointment with a female doctor or the practice nurse.
- if tests are not requested, she wants to know why

Debrief

Discuss how the doctor could, if needed, improve his performance. In particular, assess whether the doctor:

- introduced himself clearly and in a friendly way
- allowed the patient to express herself and encouraged her to give a clear picture of what she was expecting? Was the consultation structured?
- having identified the patient's request, summarised it and reflected back to her?
- closed the discussion with an agreement on how to proceed?

If the call went smoothly and ran to time, did the doctor:

- avoid poorly timed questions?
- avoid repetition, which diminishes the confidence of the caller?
- deliver questions and information in a clear manner, or were explanations complicated, overlong, full of jargon and difficult to follow?
- gather sufficient information to allow a safe assessment of the problem?
- exclude the conditions requiring more urgent action?
- negotiate an action plan?

Test your theoretical knowledge

For each of the following statements, answer true (T) or false (F).

Regarding secondary amenorrhoea (that is, the absence of menstruation for 6 consecutive months in a woman who has previously had regular periods)

1. Enquire about galactorrhoea, hirsutism, symptoms of thyroid disease, weight loss or gain, emotional upsets, exercise level, medication, and family history.
2. In resistant ovary syndrome, the ovaries contain many primordial follicles which are resistant to the action of insulin.
3. Except for prolactinomas, which usually require surgery, other tumours of the pituitary or hypothalamus commonly shrink with medical therapy.
4. Consider oestrogen replacement in women with hyperprolactinaemia because they are oestrogen-deficient and at risk of osteoporosis.
5. In a woman with amenorrhoea, estradiol levels are very useful in assessing the degree of oestrogen deficiency.
6. Prolactin levels may be moderately and more permanently elevated as a result of polycystic ovary syndrome (PCOS).
7. The investigation for Asherman's syndrome is a hysteroscopy.

Relevant literature

www.cks.library.nhs.uk/amenorrhoea#

Mock case 6 – Child with constipation

Brief to the doctor

The mother of EP, aged 4 years, wishes to consult you to discuss her daughter's bowel problem.

Patient summary

Name	EP
Date of birth (Age)	Age 4 years 1 month
Social and Family History	Only child
Past medical history	Nil of note Fully vaccinated
Current medication	Nil
Investigations	None

Tasks for the doctor

In this case, the tasks are to:
- clarify EP's problem
- develop a management plan

Brief to the patient – more about the patient

1. Profile:

- EP is aged 4 years 1 month
- she is a fit healthy happy girl who has had no significant health problems in the past
- her mother is concerned that EP has been suffering from constipation for the past 4 months because:
  - she has 2–3 bowel movements a week
  - she appears to hang on rather than go to the toilet
  - she often complains it hurts when she defaecates
  - her stools are large and hard and almost block the toilet
  - most days her underwear is stained with faeces
- EP is due to start school in a few months and her mother is very concerned that smelling of faeces due to the soiling will cause problems with other children

2. She is seeing the doctor today because:

- she would like reassurance that EP does not have a pathological cause of her symptoms
- she would like treatment to restore a normal bowel habit

3. Additional information:

- If the doctor asks specifically:
  - up until 4 months ago EP had daily bowel movements and no soiling
  - EP and her mother cannot recall any episode preceding the changed bowel habit such as passing a very painful stool, or having to hold on for a long time
  - EP has never passed any blood and only ever defecates in the toilet
  - there do not appear to be any problems at home or at EP's nursery
- the mother has talked about the problem with the nursery staff who suggested increasing EP's dietary fibre and encouraging her to drink more fluids – EP eats healthily and is not a 'fussy eater'
- EP appears to be a happy child to both her mother and to the nursery staff
- there is no family history of constipation

Debrief

This case tests the doctor's ability to:
- establish a diagnosis
- develop a management plan
- support and educate the mother

Discuss how the doctor could, if needed, improve his performance. In particular, assess whether the doctor:
- structured the consultation
- used the available time appropriately
- established the development of the condition
- identified the mother's anxieties about there being a pathological cause for EP's constipation and reassured her appropriately
- explored the social effects of EP's condition – soiling daily and about to start school
- reassured the mother and developed an agreed management plan
- encouraged lifestyle changes such as diet change
- discussed star charts
- prescribed laxatives appropriately
- arranged follow-up
- considered involving other members of the PCT such as the Health Visitor or School Nurse
- safety-netted by advising about side-effects of laxatives and clarifying when to seek help earlier than planned

Test your theoretical knowledge

For each of the following statements, answer true (T) or false (F).

1. Constipation is one of the 10 most common problems seen by general paediatricians
2. A plain abdominal X-ray should always be taken as part of the initial assessment to exclude a rectal faecal mass
3. Osmotic laxatives are not recommended
4. Prolonged use of stimulant laxatives can cause hypokalaemia
5. 98% of children are toilet trained by the age of 4 years

Relevant literature

Rubin G, Dale A. (2006) Chronic constipation in children. *BMJ,* **333:** 1051–1055.

Mock case 7 – Problem drinking

Brief to the doctor

Mr MS is a 26 year old man who has consulted in the past for various rugby injuries. He presents today sporting a few facial injuries.

Patient summary

Name	MS
Date of birth (Age)	26
Social and Family History	Unmarried Works for a logistics company Plays front row for the local amateur rugby club
Past medical history	Hayfever (every spring) Acne vulgaris (4 months ago) Left AC joint injury (5 months ago) Right ACL reconstruction (2 years ago)
Past medication	Loratidine 10 mg daily (spring) Minocycline 100 mg twice daily (4 months ago)

Tasks for the doctor

In this case, the tasks are to:
- assess an individual patient's risk factors
- demonstrate an understanding of the concept of risk and be able to communicate risk effectively and sensitively to the patient
- negotiate a shared understanding of the problem and its management (including self-management) with the patient, so that the patient is empowered to self-care
- demonstrate skills to transform holistic understanding of the presenting problem into practical measures to move the patient forward

Brief to the patient – more about the patient

1. Profile:

- Mr MS is a 26 year old man who has worked at the local logistics company since leaving school
- he is a good rugby player and his social life revolves around the rugby club
- he is unmarried but has been in a steady relationship for 11 months
- his girlfriend is attending the local teacher training college and her family live 2 hours drive away
- his older brother married young (age 19) and divorced 3 years later. He has experienced difficulty in seeing his children. Mr MS's mother often says she feels sad that her grandchildren *"are strangers to her"*.

2. He is seeing the doctor today because:

- he wants a referral to the practice counsellor for *"help with my drinking"*
- he says that his drinking has increased over the last 6 weeks and he has been in trouble twice with the police
- on these two occasions, he got into fights while drunk and the police became involved; on the last occasion he had to be restrained, hence the bruises on his face
- the police hearings are set for a week and a month away; the police have told him that he *"is throwing his life and career away"*, so he is heeding their advice and is now seeking help
- the fights were unprovoked; nobody was seriously injured because he *"loses all coordination when drunk"*
- when asked what he is angry with, he says *"with life and circumstances"*. His girlfriend is 4 months pregnant with his child. He feels uncertain about getting married and says he is too young to become a father. He feels angry about the contraception failure.
- his girlfriend plans to move in with him into his parents' house because they cannot afford to live on their own. His parents have been supportive. Although he hasn't decided to marry yet, he feels his mum will become attached to the baby and it will be difficult to part ways after the baby's birth.
- his girlfriend, after the last fight, asked if he wanted her to move out – they are working things through
- he usually binges after rugby matches, but restricts his intake to less than 20 units per week; over the last 6 weeks, he has been drinking *"way more than this"* and tries to pass out so he doesn't have to think about his situation
- his main symptom is anxiety about his future – he does not have symptoms of depression
- he would like to speak to someone *"to sort out my head"* and he expects a referral to the practice counsellor

3. Additional information:

- if the doctor discusses Alcoholics Anonymous with him, he says he is not an alcoholic and doesn't think their service is appropriate to his needs
- if signposted to local services (Relate or social services), he wants to know how these services could be useful to him
- if you arrange follow-up, he wants to know when and why he should attend

Debrief

Discuss how the doctor could, if needed, improve his performance. In particular, assess whether the doctor:

- explored the problem using open and closed questions? Was time allowed for the patient to think before answering?
- facilitated the patient's responses and clarified statements that were unclear (e.g. *"Could you explain what you mean by trouble with the police"*)
- determined the patient's ideas (cause of his anger), concerns (not feeling ready for fatherhood), and expectations (a counsellor with whom he could discuss feelings and issues)
- used empathy to communicate an understanding of the patient's predicament
- gave an explanation or demonstrated support at appropriate times? Did the doctor avoid giving advice or reassurance prematurely?
- involved the patient by making suggestions rather than issuing directives? Was the patient's view of need for action, perceived benefits, barriers, and motivation assessed?
- closed by summarising the consultation briefly and clarifying his plan of care?

If the consultation over-ran, did the doctor:
- take a structured history that explored the problem drinking holistically?
- insist on selling certain managements options, such as Alcoholics Anonymous instead of negotiating with the patient?
- perform unnecessary examinations?

Test your theoretical knowledge

For each of the following statements, answer true (T) or false (F).

Regarding problem drinking
1. Asking a person how much alcohol they drink has a high sensitivity for diagnosing an alcohol problem
2. The association between signs (tremor of the hands and tongue, and excessive capillarisation of the skin and conjunctivae) and increased alcohol intake has been thoroughly investigated
3. Appropriate screening helps to detect and treat alcohol problems
4. The CAGE questionnaire is more sensitive than the AUDIT questionnaire in detecting hazardous drinking
5. Biochemical markers can lead to false-positive results if used as a screening test, and are neither sensitive nor specific for diagnosing an alcohol problem
6. Fatty liver is present in 25% of persistently heavy drinkers
7. Aim for moderation, rather than abstinence, in people who are drinking hazardous amounts of alcohol, who do not have overt signs of physical or psychological harm

Relevant literature

www.sign.ac.uk/pdf/sign74.pdf

People should be signposted to agencies that can provide practical advice and help to manage the problems. Agencies include:

- counselling services (in the GP practice or locally) for anxiety, depression, and relationship counselling
- Citizens Advice for financial, housing, or employment problems (see www.citizensadvice.org.uk)
- Alcohol Concern for general information (see www.alcoholconcern.org.uk)
- Alcoholics Anonymous mainly for dependence, but also provides help for family members (see www.alcoholics-anonymous.org.uk)

Mock case 8 – Lower abdominal pain

Brief to the doctor

Mrs KN is a 35 year old woman who has been booked into your surgery as an emergency. She presents with per vaginal (PV) bleeding and lower abdominal pain.

Patient summary

Name	KN
Date of birth (Age)	35
Social and Family History	Married 2 years ago. No children Book-keeper at a local company
Past medical history	Pre-pregnancy counselling (2 weeks ago) Irritable bowel syndrome (1 month ago)
Past medication	Mebeverine 135 mg thrice daily × 100T (1 month ago)

Consultation note by Dr Brown (2 weeks ago):
'Stopped Microgynon 12 months ago. Then husband worked overseas for four months. So, trying for a baby for past 8 months. LMP 27 day, three months ago. Missed last two periods and then has a bleed lasting 24 hours. Two pregnancy tests last month were negative. Recent blood tests, including hormone profile, were fine. Plan: get 21 day progestogen. In view of age (and husband is 38; neither have had children) refer to fertility clinic at next appointment.'

Tasks for the doctor

In this case, the tasks are to:
- be able to prioritise problems and establish a differential diagnosis
- make the patient's safety a priority
- consider the appropriateness of interventions according to patient's wishes, the severity of the illness and any chronic or co-morbid diseases
- recognise patients who are likely to need acute care and offer them advice on prevention, effective self-management and when and who to call for help

Brief to the patient – more about the patient

1. Profile:

- Mrs KN is a 35 year old woman who works as a book-keeper at a local company
- she is a fit and healthy – she runs 5 miles two to three times per week
- she is married to a multinational employee, aged 38, and he occasionally works overseas – he returned from a 4-month stint in the Middle East 8 months ago
- she is an only child and her elderly parents live in the North East of England

2. She is seeing the doctor today because:

- she has had right iliac fossa and suprapubic pain for 3 days
- the pain is intermittent, with spasms that develop, reach a peak (8/10), and then subside to a dull ache; this pattern has occurred every few hours for the last 3 days and seems to be getting worse, rather than better
- it does not feel like her usual IBS pain
- the only associated symptom is PV bleeding, which started 20 days ago; initially she assumed this was her period, but the bleeding, though light, has continued – her usual cycle is 6/30
- she does not have urinary frequency, dysuria, diarrhoea or vomiting; she has eaten today.
- she thinks *"something is wrong"* and suspects appendicitis or a miscarriage
- she is worried about having a miscarriage. Her husband is in a meeting in Belfast and she is worried about calling him and disrupting his meeting if she only has a minor ailment. On the other hand, she is scared about having a miscarriage or being admitted into hospital without him.
- she expects to be told her diagnosis, prognosis and treatment plan. She wants sufficient information to decide whether she should ask her husband to shorten his business trip and return home tonight.
- her main symptoms are pelvic pain for 3 ½ days and light PV bleeding for 20 days; she does not feel pregnant
- when she saw Dr Brown 2 weeks ago, she was advised to have a blood test 7 days before her next period was due but because she was missing periods, she didn't know when to come in for the test, so the test was not done.

3. Additional information:

- if the doctor asks to test her urine, she produces a piece of paper: Urine pregnancy test positive. Dipstix: trace leucocytes but no nitrites or protein.

- if the doctor offers to perform a pelvic examination, she declines. Unless there are compelling reasons for the examination, she declines to be examined while bleeding.
- if the doctor says he will phone the gynaecologist on call to arrange an urgent review, she produces a slip of paper: *"Gynae registrar on call arranged for an emergency scan at 09h00 tomorrow in OPD. Patient advised to attend A&E if pain worsens or she becomes unwell"*

Debrief

This case was written about a woman presenting with an ectopic pregnancy. Her social support is minimal. The doctor needs to suspect an ectopic pregnancy, broach the possibility of bad news, support her and deal with the emergency.

Discuss how the doctor could, if needed, improve his performance. In particular, assess whether the doctor:

- identified the patient's problem with an appropriate opening question, e.g. *"What can I do for you today?"*
- established dates and sequence of events
- encouraged the patient to express her feelings?
- demonstrated appropriate confidence?
- assessed the patient's prior knowledge before giving information and gave explanations after discovering the extent of patient's wish for information?
- checked with the patient whether plans were accepted and if concerns were addressed
- explained seriousness, expected outcome, short and long term consequences?
- safety netted by explaining possible unexpected outcomes and clarified when and how to seek help?

If the consultation over-ran:

- was the doctor repetitive and disorganised in his history taking?
- were unnecessary examinations attempted, failing to take into account the patient's wishes?
- was the doctor unable to establish a differential diagnosis, recognise the need for further investigation and arrange for appropriate help within the allocated time?

Test your theoretical knowledge

For each of the following statements, answer true (T) or false (F).

Regarding ectopic pregnancies

1. Cramping period-like pains and slight vaginal bleeding usually occur between weeks 4 and 10 of pregnancy
2. Shoulder tip pain or diarrhoea or blood in the stools are symptoms of ectopic pregnancy
3. If the pregnancy is very early, the ectopic might not be clear on the first transabdominal scan, so a second scan is done a few days later
4. Most ectopic pregnancies require sudden emergency treatment rather than planned, urgent surgery
5. Methotrexate is licensed for the treatment of early ectopic pregnancy

Relevant literature

http://cks.library.nhs.uk/patient_information_leaflet/ectopic_pregnancy/introduction#-277427

Mock case 9 – Hypertension

Brief to the doctor

Mr GM is a 47 year old man who has been referred to you by the practice nurse for a medical review of his hypertension.

Patient summary

Name	GM
Date of birth (Age)	47
Social and Family History	Divorced, with one teenage son
	Works as a telecommunications engineer
Past medical history	Saw physiotherapist for cervicalgia (8 months ago)
	Hypertension (2 years)
Repeat medication	Perindopril 4 mg od × 28T

Consultation note by practice nurse (2 weeks ago):

'Routine BP check. Mum and sister have HT. Alcohol consumption 24 units per week. Never smoked tobacco. Thinks high BP today may be due to recent work stresses. Plan: Get U&Es. May need change in medication, so will do home readings and see GP with results.'

Blood tests	Tests were done 2 weeks ago
Sodium	137 mmol/l (135–145)
Potassium	4.2 mmol/l (3.5–5)
Creatinine	118 umol/l (70–150)
Urea	6.6 mmol/l (2.5–6.7)
BP	131/ 97 and 141/91
BMI	31.1
	Tests from 2 years ago
Fasting glucose	5.1 mmol/l (3–5.5)
Total cholesterol	4.9 mmol/l
HDL	1.23 mmol/l
ECG	LVH by voltage criteria
BP	129/85 and 124/86

Tasks for the doctor

In this case, the tasks are to:

- identify the patient's health beliefs regarding cardiovascular disease and either reinforce, modify or challenge these beliefs as appropriate
- recognise that non-concordance is common for many preventative cardiovascular medicines and respect the patient's autonomy when negotiating management
- communicate the patient's risk of cardiovascular problems clearly and effectively in a non-biased manner

Brief to the patient – more about the patient

1. Profile:

- Mr GM is a 47 year old man. He is a senior telecommunication engineer. His current work is mainly office based. He is worried about job cuts and salary reductions as the company is going through a lean period.
- He divorced 2 years ago. His teenage son, who is taking A-levels, chose to live with him to attend the local school. He is now in a new relationship and would like to marry his partner. However, he is waiting until his son moves to university before selling his house and moving in with his partner. He is not getting on well with his son at present.

2. He is seeing the doctor today because:

- he wants to know the results of his recent blood tests; the practice nurse told him he may need to increase his blood pressure medication but he's not too keen on taking more pills
- he does not want to take more medicines because he thinks his BP readings may be due to 'stress', both at home and at work; he thinks he should continue with his current medication and exercise a bit more
- he has not done the home readings as advised by the nurse because he forgot to loan out the BP machine from the practice – he thought you could check his BP today
- several issues cause 'stress': his teenage son seems more interested in his social life than in studying and may not get a place at university. He is worried about delaying putting his house on the market and now house prices are falling. There have been talks about salary reductions at work.
- he talks about doing more exercise but, when challenged, is unable to identify when he will find time to exercise. He already feels rushed and because he feels tired, he eats more ready-made meals and has increased his alcohol intake. He admits to missing the occasional BP pill.
- he is asymptomatic from his hypertension and does not experience any untoward side effects from medication; he expects to get a repeat prescription of his BP medication and to return for a nurse review in six months

3. Additional information:

- if the doctor takes his BP today, it is 140/90 and, if repeated, 142/89
- if the doctor discusses changing his BP medication, he wants to know the advantages and disadvantages with this course of action; he is afraid of side effects such as erectile dysfunction and lethargy
- if exercise and diet are discussed, he says he will try to do more but fails to identify how he will convert his good intentions into action
- if compliance is discussed, he says he keeps his tablets at his house and therefore does not take them when he stays over at his partner's place

Debrief

Discuss how the doctor could, if needed, improve his performance. In particular, assess whether the doctor:

- actively and appropriately explored the patient's ideas (his belief about the effect of stress on BP); his concerns (worries about potential drug side effects); his expectations (of deferring medication changes to a later date when his personal circumstances are less stressful)
- encouraged Mr GM to express his feelings and was non-judgemental when listening
- provided concise and easily understood explanations
- involved the patient by making suggestions rather than issuing directives
- encouraged a discussion about potential anxieties
- encouraged Mr GM to take responsibility

If the consultation was too short, did the doctor:
- fail to identify and address the psycho-social issues affecting Mr GM's treatment?
- address the issue of partial compliance?
- address the treatment of hypertension to acceptable targets using add-on medication in line with NICE guidance?

Test your theoretical knowledge

For each of the following statements, answer true (T) or false (F).

Regarding hypertension
1. Where patients do not have the capacity to make decisions about their hypertensive treatments, healthcare professionals should follow the advice in 'Reference guide to consent for examination or treatment' (DoH)
2. Routine use of home monitoring devices in primary care is recommended; their value has been adequately established
3. Offer drug therapy to patients at raised cardiovascular risk (10-year risk of CVD of 15% or more, or existing CVD or target organ damage) with persistent blood pressure of more than 140/90 mmHg
4. In black and Asian patients, the first choice for initial therapy should be either a calcium-channel blocker or a thiazide-type diuretic
5. If the first measurement exceeds 140/90 mmHg, if practical, take a second confirmatory reading at the end of the consultation
6. A fall in systolic BP when standing of 20 mmHg or more indicates postural hypotension

Relevant literature

www.nice.org.uk/nicemedia/pdf/CG034NICEguideline.doc

www.rcgp-curriculum.org.uk/PDF/curr_15_1_Cardiovascular_problems.pdf

www.gp-training.net/training/communication_skills/calgary/ice.htm

Mock case 10 – Abdominal symptoms

Brief to the doctor

Mr RF is a 32 year old man with continuing abdominal symptoms following elimination therapy for *H. pylori*.

Patient summary

Name	RF
Date of birth (Age)	32
Social and Family History	Married with one child (2 years old) Works as an electrical appliance engineer
Past medical history	Abdominal pain (6 months ago)
Past medication	Triple therapy for *H. pylori* (6 months ago)

Consultation note by Dr Brown (6 months ago):
'Worried about loose stool, thrice daily x 2 weeks, since return from holiday. Stool has "always been loose" but frequency is new and not controlled by immodium. Also painful tongue. No dyspepsia symptoms but recent H. pylori *serology is positive. Never had treatment for this in past. FBC, CRP and LFTs are normal. Plan: treat with triple therapy. If no response to treatment, then refer to gastroenterology.'*

Blood tests	Tests were done 6 months ago
FBC	no abnormalities
ESR	8 mm/h
Urea and electrolytes	no abnormalities
Liver function tests	no abnormalities
H. pylori serology	positive

Tasks for the doctor

In this case, the tasks are to:

- demonstrate the knowledge, skills and attitudes for effective communication in eliciting and understanding the values of patients, negotiating an acceptable course of action and justifying that course of action
- integrate knowledge of the patient's values with the relevant scientific evidence and clinical experience to achieve the best outcome for the patient
- practise holistically by enabling the patient to make choices about how he wishes to live his life by exploring what is important to the patient overall and not restricting information-sharing to clinical data

Brief to the patient – more about the patient

1. Profile:

- Mr RF is a 32 year old married man
- he works as an electrical appliance engineer for a local company; he is planning to set up his own business soon, having acquired the relevant skills, qualifications and experience from his current job
- he is married to JF, aged 35, and they have one son; they have a good relationship. JF has not returned to work as a nursery assistant since the birth of their son and he is the sole breadwinner.
- he is optimistic but slightly anxious about starting his own business

2. He is seeing the doctor today because:

- he looked up his symptoms (loose stool, abdominal discomfort, tiredness, diarrhoea and painful tongue) on the internet and thinks he may have coeliac disease; he wants your opinion regarding diagnosis, tests and treatments
- he does not have joint pains, skin problems, night sweats or weight loss
- his mother has had bowel problems for a long time but he hasn't discussed his symptoms with her – *"she is a hypochondriac"*
- his bowel symptoms improved while he was on triple therapy but returned the moment he completed the course. He does not think he had dyspepsia; he told Dr Brown this but she was adamant that the positive *H. pylori* serology warranted treatment. He wants to know if you think that Dr Brown *"got it wrong?"*
- he has stopped eating gluten for 3 weeks and feels much better – this weekend, he ate a hamburger bun and felt unwell
- the gluten exclusion and re-challenge has convinced him that he has coeliac disease. He is concerned that the diagnosis has been missed. He is also concerned about the effect a positive diagnosis may have on the insurance he needs to take out when he becomes a self-employed tradesman. He expects to be told about what investigations are needed, and whether he should delay testing until after his insurance medical. If he delays testing, he asks what you will write on his medical form?

3. Additional information:

- if the doctor discusses further investigation with him, he requests information about the predictive value of the tests and specifically asks about *"a bowel biopsy"*
- if the doctor arranges for blood tests, he wants to know when these should be done and whether he should remain off gluten until testing occurs
- he specifically wants to know what you will write on his insurance medical forms before or after his investigations – if you were him, would you delay investigations until after the insurance medical?

Debrief

Discuss how the doctor could, if needed, improve his performance. In particular, assess whether the doctor:

- demonstrated an interest in the patient's presenting issues, that is, did the doctor listen attentively and explore problems using a mix of open and closed questions
- respected the patient's attempt to make sense of his symptoms using information from the internet – this could be gauged from the doctor's non-verbal behaviour (eye contact, facial expression, posture, and rate/ volume/ tone of speech)
- shared his thinking with the patient to encourage his involvement (e.g. *"What I'm thinking of in terms of further testing is ...."*)
- assessed the patient's prior knowledge before giving information and gave sufficient information to address his specific concerns and expectations
- shared his own thinking on the insurance dilemma with the patient and behaved professionally and ethically
- closed by summarising the session briefly and clarifying the management plan

If the consultation over-ran, did the doctor:
- take a history in a systematic, logical and structured manner?
- provide explanations in a logical and concise manner?
- duplicate information the patient already had from his internet reading?
- address irrelevant issues?

Test your theoretical knowledge

For each of the following statements, answer true (T) or false (F).

Regarding coeliac disease
1. It is an autoimmune condition triggered in genetically predisposed individuals by the consumption of gluten
2. Coeliac disease characteristically causes inflammatory changes in the ascending colon; however, any organ system can be affected
3. Patients report diarrhoea, constipation, nausea or reflux as symptoms
4. Serological testing and duodenal biopsy should be the first investigations
5. False positive serology occurs in 5–10% of cases with anti-endomysial antibodies (EmA) and for anti-transglutaminase antibodies (TGA) using human recombinant antigen
6. Negative antibody tests do not preclude positive serology and development of coeliac disease in the future
7. As people medically diagnosed with coeliac disease cannot eat foods made from wheat flour, special gluten-free bread, flour mixes, pasta, pizza bases, biscuits and crackers are available on prescription

Relevant literature

www.crestni.org.uk/publications/coeliac-disease-adult-diagnosis.pdf

Mock case 11 – Allergy symptoms

Brief to the doctor

Mrs RW is a 33 year old woman who has come to talk to you about her son's skin problems, which she believes are due to cow's milk allergy. She is also upset with Dr Brown whom she saw about this problem last week.

Patient summary

Name	Oliver W
Date of birth (Age)	5 months
Social and Family History	His parents are married and he is an only child Dad is a secondary school English teacher; mum is a librarian
Past medical history	Infantile eczema (since birth)
Repeat medication	Epaderm ointment qds × 500 g Oilatum plus bath emollient – 1 cupful in bath × 500 ml Hydrocortisone 1% as directed × 15 g

Consultation note by Dr Brown (1 week ago):
'Comes out in some sort of urticarial reaction wherever formula milk touches his skin. Mainly breast-fed. O/E: nothing to see today. Plan: as no GI upset with the milk, try Wysol.'

Tasks for the doctor

In this case, the tasks are to:
- manage conditions which may present early and in an undifferentiated way
- achieve concordance with mum, including active listening and shared decision-making
- coordinate care with other primary care professionals, paediatricians and other appropriate specialists, leading to effective and appropriate care provision, taking an advocacy position for the patient or family when needed

Brief to the patient – more about the patient

1. Profile:

- Mrs RW is a 33 year old woman who, on completion of her maternity leave in 3 months, intends to return to work as a part-time librarian at the university
- Oliver is 5 months old; he was born at 36 weeks by emergency caesarean section for a breech presentation
- Oliver was breast-fed from birth; mum is trying to introduce one bottle of formula at night but has run into problems
- Oliver has gained weight well since birth, is just below the 50th centile and is developing well
- two months ago he presented with dry skin on his trunk and face, diagnosed as eczema; dad's brother had childhood eczema
- Oliver is up to date with childhood immunisations

2. His mum is seeing the doctor today because:

- she is unhappy with last week's consultation with Dr Brown – she feels her concerns about possible cow's milk allergy were dismissed and soya milk was prescribed inappropriately
- she suspects cow's milk allergy because after her consultation with Dr Brown, she went home, placed some formula on Oliver's skin and within an hour, he developed an angry red patch. She was upset; she called in her neighbour, a nurse, to help (and witness) Oliver's reactions. They washed off the formula but the skin took 12 hours to return to normal. In the past, little dribbles of formula onto the skin around his mouth produced angry red patches and caused his eczema to flare.
- she is concerned about the safety of soya milk. According to her internet reading, soya milk should not be prescribed to children under 1 year. Should she give the soya milk, as prescribed by Dr Brown?
- she expects you to refer Oliver to the paediatric allergy clinic. She would like advice on weaning, particularly which fruit or vegetables she should avoid. She also wants to know whether she should continue drinking cow's milk while breast-feeding.

3. Additional information:

- if the doctor asks about allergies in the family, she says her husband develops nettle rash if he eats papaya; neither parent is atopic
- if asked about her health beliefs, she thinks that Oliver's mild eczema has deteriorated because of his allergy to cows' milk
- if asked what she would like to do about her unhappiness with Dr Brown, she says she wants to lodge a written complaint and expects information about the practice complaint's system

Debrief

Discuss how the doctor could, if needed, improve his performance. In particular, assess whether the doctor:

- identified, at the outset, the issues the parent wished to address today, perhaps with an appropriate opening question such as *"What can I do for you today?"*
- facilitated the parent's responses either verbally or non-verbally, for example, was the patient encouraged; were Mrs RW's words repeated, paraphrased or interpreted?
- addressed Mrs RW's ideas (that there is link between cows' milk allergy and eczema), concerns (about the safety of soya milk in children under 1 year and her dairy intake while breast-feeding), and expectations (for referral to allergy clinic and signposting to the practice complaint's procedure)
- expressed concern, understanding, and a willingness to help
- provided clear information on procedures and management plans

If the consultation over-ran, did the doctor:

- spend a disproportionate amount of time on the data-gathering without moving fluently into the explanation/management part of the consultation?
- flounder when negotiating management plans, perhaps due to a lack of knowledge about the clinical presentation or the complaints system?
- have a dysfunctional consultation because he'd initially failed either to create rapport or to address the parent's specific ideas, concerns and expectations?

Test your theoretical knowledge

For each of the following statements, answer true (T) or false (F).

Regarding cows' milk allergy
1. Cows' milk allergy, after egg allergy, is the 2nd most common food allergy in childhood
2. It is more common in babies with atopic dermatitis
3. Babies with cows' milk allergy can react to milk protein from breast milk, from cows' milk, or formula based on cows' milk
4. Half the children who have an allergy to cows' milk will still be allergic to it as adults
5. The symptoms of milk allergy include rashes, diarrhoea, vomiting, stomach cramps and difficulty in breathing
6. The allergic reaction is to whey, not casein
7. Heat treatment, such as pasteurisation, changes whey, so people who are sensitive to whey are unlikely to react to pasteurised milk
8. Heat treatment affects casein, so someone who is allergic to casein is unlikely to react to pasteurised milk

Relevant literature

www.eatwell.gov.uk/healthissues/foodintolerance/foodintolerancetypes/milkallergy/

Mock case 12 – Late for depo-provera

Brief to the doctor

Mrs CA is a 22 year old woman who has recently joined your practice. She presents 15 weeks and 5 days since her last depo-provera injection.

Patient summary

Name	CA
Date of birth (Age)	22
Social and Family History	Married on the day her depo-provera injection was due (3 weeks + 5 days ago) Currently looking for work locally; waitressing
Past medical history	Nil significant
Past medication	Medroxyprogesterone acetate 150 mg / 1ml × 1 injection given 15 weeks and 5 days ago

Tasks for the doctor

In this case, the tasks are to:
- advise and provide suitable methods for family planning
- provide sufficient information to move the consultation forward
- involve the patient in the management plan

Brief to the patient – more about the patient

1. Profile:

- Mrs CA is a 22 year old woman who married a local man recently and moved to the area; she is new to the practice
- she used to work as receptionist at a garage sales company and is currently looking for office work; she waitresses at the moment
- she wants to start her family in 3–5 years; until then, she wants to do a bit of travelling
- she is slightly concerned about finding a new job; *"waiting tables won't fund interesting and exotic holidays"*
- her sister has recently returned from New Zealand; Mrs CA would like to walk the Milford Sound trail in the next year

2. She is seeing the doctor today because:

- she knows she is late for her depo and needs contraception
- the depo was due on the day of her wedding. She remembered when she returned from her honeymoon (2 weeks in Barcelona) and called the practice – the receptionist told her the next available family planning appointment was today (5 days after telephoning)
- since the depo 'ran out' on her wedding day, she and her husband have used condoms; she had 'an accident' last week but cannot remember exactly which day, but it was definitely more than 3 days ago
- the pregnancy test she did last week, the morning after the accident, was negative
- she wants depo contraception today; she does not want the Pill; she chokes on them – *"it's a mental thing"*
- she is interested in long-acting contraception, particularly implanon. She heard that it could take quite long to get pregnant after discontinuing depo.
- she does not have risk factors for osteoporosis and has no contra-indications to hormonal contraception

3. Additional information:

- if the doctor discusses urine pregnancy testing, she wants to know how long it takes for these tests to become positive
- if the doctor discusses giving depo (or inserting the implant or IUS) today, she wants to know if there are any consequences to a potential pregnancy
- if the doctor discusses deferring the contraception until 3 weeks after the unprotected sex, she is unhappy with this; she says her husband is getting fed up with condoms
- if the doctor discusses emergency contraception, she wants to know its efficacy
- if offered depo, she takes it

Debrief

Discuss how the doctor could, if needed, improve his performance. In particular, assess whether the doctor:

- established the dates and sequence of events
- appropriately explored and addressed the patient's ideas (beliefs about pregnancy testing the day after unprotected sex), concerns (worries about her husband discontinuing condom use), and expectations (help with obtaining timely family planning advice)
- gave information about pregnancy testing, emergency contraception and long-acting contraception in assimilable chunks and checked for understanding after each piece of information was imparted
- organised his explanation into discrete sections
- discussed options and negotiated a mutually acceptable plan
- safety-netted

If the consultation over-ran, did the doctor:

- muddle up dates and fail to establish the sequence of events?
- provide complicated and long explanations without stopping to check understanding?
- fail to address the patient's expectation of obtaining suitable and effective family planning?

Test your theoretical knowledge

For each of the following statements, answer true (T) or false (F).

Regarding contraception

1. Two consecutive doses of combined oral contraceptive are required to inhibit ovulation; subsequent doses maintain anovulation
2. Progestogen-only pills (POPs), containing norgestrel, desogestrel, levonorgestrel, norethisterone, or etynodiol diacetate, work by thinning cervical mucus, increasing ovum transport, inhibiting ovulation, and providing an endometrium hostile to implantation
3. The formulations of depot medroxyprogesterone acetate and nerethisterone enantate slowly release the active components and provide effective therapeutic levels for 12 weeks
4. Serum etonogestrel concentrations rise rapidly after insertion of the implant, and ovulation is likely to be inhibited within 24 hours
5. The copper IUD can work immediately after insertion
6. Few women (< 25%) will continue to ovulate while using the levonorgestrel-releasing intrauterine system (IUS)
7. The efficacy of female condoms in preventing transmission of hepatitis A, B, and C is unknown

Relevant literature

http://cks.library.nhs.uk/contraception/leaflets_for_patients/contraceptive_
injections_your_guide_fpa/contraceptive_injections_your_guide/how_does_depo_
provera_affect_my_bones

Mock case 13 - Raised cholesterol

Brief to the doctor

Mr CB is a 46 year old man who had blood tests undertaken two weeks ago. He returns to discuss the results. He also has a 2nd issue on which he'd like advice.

Patient summary

Name   CB

Date of birth (Age)   46

Social and Family History   Has two sons (age 14 and 12 years) and one daughter (6 years)
                                  Is a computer software engineer

Past medical history   Tennis elbow (4 years ago)

Consultation note by Dr Brown (4 weeks ago):
'Informed about last week's tests – cholesterol slightly high. Mum was recently diagnosed with type 2 DM (diet controlled). No other family risk factors for IHD. 10 cig per day – smoking cessation advised. Doing 3 x 45 minute gym workouts and lost 4 kg since Christmas. O/E: 137/89. BMI 28.1. Plan: get repeat bloods and review in 4–6 weeks.'

Blood tests   Repeat tests were done 1 week ago
  Total cholesterol   6.3 mmol/l
  HDL   1.0 mmol/l (0.8–1.8 U)
  Plasma triglyceride   2.81 mmol/l (0.55–1.9 U)
  TSH   4.28 µM/l (0.35–5.5)

                                  Tests done 5 weeks ago
  Total cholesterol   6.2 mmol/l
  HDL   0.9 mmol/l (0.8–1.8 U)
  Plasma triglyceride   2.81 mmol/l (0.55–1.9 U)
  Fasting glucose   5.3 (3–5.5 U)
  Liver function tests   normal
  Renal function tests   normal

Tasks for the doctor

In this case, the tasks are to:

- communicate risk effectively to the patient
- describe the effects of smoking and hypercholesterolaemia on the patient and his family
- help the patient understand work–life balance and, where appropriate, help him achieve a good work–life balance

Brief to the patient – more about the patient

1. Profile:

- Mr CB is a 46 year old married man with three children; the two boys are weekly boarders in public school
- he works as a software engineer at a large multinational company where his job involves travel, in the UK and overseas; he usually spends weekends and one week night at home; the rest is spent in hotels
- he eats most meals in restaurants on the company expense account. He drinks with colleagues. When he drinks, he smokes. He tries to restrict smoking to less than 10 cigarettes per week. He has smoked on and off for 18 years.
- a lot of time is spent travelling; he reads, watches television and tries to walk with his family at weekends

2. He is seeing the doctor today because:

- he wants to know the results of his recent blood tests – both sets were fasting tests
- he wants to know how the raised cholesterol affects him and whether tablet treatment is needed
- one of his wife's 'arty' friends suggested garlic – what do you think?
- he is asymptomatic; his job is stressful, mainly because of the travel and politics, *"but whose isn't"*
- his wife is concerned about his health. One of their friends recently had a heart attack at age 49. His wife thinks he needs to live a healthier life, stop smoking and lose weight but she doesn't realise how difficult this is when four nights out of seven are spent eating hotel food and grabbing a bite on the motorway. He needs his job to maintain his affluent lifestyle.
- His second issue is that his 6 year old daughter was diagnosed with hand, foot and mouth disease this week – is she OK to visit her aunt who is 24 weeks pregnant?

3. Additional information:

- if the doctor discusses lifestyle modification with him, he wants to know how he can incorporate these changes into his hectic lifestyle
- if the doctor discusses statins with him, he wants to know the risks and benefits of treatment
- if smoking cessation is offered, he says he cannot commit to the fortnightly nurse appointments; do you offer late opening hours on a Friday or Saturday morning appointments?

Debrief

Discuss how the doctor could, if needed, improve his performance. In particular, assess whether the doctor:

- was able to assess, interpret and explain Mr CB's risk factors? If so, which questions and explanations were useful?
- interpreted the evidence about primary prevention and applied this knowledge to Mr CB
- maintained an holistic approach and promoted self-care
- appropriately involved relevant members of the primary healthcare team in health promotion
- empowered the patient and involved him in the management plan

If the consultation over-ran, did the doctor:

- make offers Mr CB continued to reject instead of seeking solutions from Mr CB?
- provide complicated explanations about cholesterol and statins?
- fail to provide information about numbers needed to treat in a manner that Mr CB was able to understand?
- attempt to deal with issues the patient had not prioritised and which the doctor felt could safely wait until the next review?

Test your theoretical knowledge

For each of the following statements, answer true (T) or false (F).

Regarding lipid modification

1. Treatment for the primary and secondary prevention of CVD should be initiated with simvastatin 20 mg
2. Opportunistic assessment should be the main strategy used in primary care to identify CVD risk in unselected people
3. The Framingham risk equation should be used for people with familial hypercholesterolaemia and type 2 diabetes
4. The estimated CVD risk should be increased by a factor of 1.5 in people with a first-degree relative with a history of CHD before the age of 55
5. People at high risk of, or with, CVD should be advised to consume at least two portions of fish per week, including a portion of oily fish
6. People at high risk of, or with, CVD should be advised to take 25 minutes of physical activity a day, of at least moderate intensity, at least 3 days a week
7. A target for total or LDL cholesterol is not recommended for people who are treated with a statin for primary prevention of CVD
8. Once a person has been started on a statin for primary prevention, repeat lipid measurement is unnecessary
9. Liver function (transaminases) should be measured within 3 months of starting treatment and at 12 months, but not again unless clinically indicated

10. Numbers needed to treat represents how many people would need to receive a particular treatment or intervention in order that one of them should benefit from the treatment

Relevant literature

www.nice.org.uk/nicemedia/pdf/CG67NICEguideline.doc

www.npci.org.uk/nsm/nsm/statins/resources/pda_Statin_9.pdf

www.nntonline.com/ebm/visualrx/what.asp – pages 3 and 4 of this provide a very useful visual interpretation of NNT

Mock case 14 – Atrial fibrillation

Brief to the doctor

Mr KV is a retired biology teacher aged 67. He saw a GP a month ago because he kept feeling his heart flutter. He was well at the time and the GP advised him to attend if his symptoms recurred.

Patient summary

Name	KV
Date of birth (Age)	67
Social and Family History	Single
Past medical history	Nil of note
Current medication	Nil
Investigations	None

Tasks for the doctor

In this case, the tasks are to:
- establish a diagnosis
- formulate a management plan

Brief to the patient – more about the patient

1. Profile:

- Mr KV is a 67 year old retired biology teacher
- he is single and lives alone
- he has enjoyed excellent health until the last few months
- he has never smoked

2. He is seeing the doctor today because:

- he started having episodes when he felt his heart flutter about 2 months ago. He saw a GP a month ago, but was well when seen. The GP told him to re-attend if his symptoms recurrred.
- his symptoms returned just before he went on a walking holiday in Scotland 3 weeks ago and have remained since
- he feels that his heart is fluttering but there is no pain; he does get slightly breathless on exertion and cannot walk as far as previously
- he is keen to have a diagnosis and be treated

3. Additional information:

- He has no history of indigestion, or asthma.
- If the doctor examines him:

System	Findings
General	Slim, healthy Urine neg. to glucose, protein, and blood
CVS	Pulse 140 irregularly irregular JVP not raised No murmur BP 138/84 No oedema
Respiratory	RR normal Chest sounds clear
Abdomen	No organomegaly No ascites

- If the doctor arranges an ECG, an ECG showing AF with a rate of 140 is produced, or a report stating 'AF Rate 140'.
- If the doctor says he would like to talk to the hospital – "*Medical registrar advises that there is no indication for acute admission, but the patient should be referred and the doctor initiate appropriate treatment in the meantime.*".
- If the doctor discusses treatment, he will want to know what the medication will do and any side effects.

Debrief

This case tests the doctor's ability to:
- integrate information from the history, examination and ECG to make a diagnosis of AF
- arrange further tests
- treat in accordance with NICE guidance

Discuss how the doctor could, if needed, improve his performance. In particular, assess whether the doctor:
- identified the patient's symptoms
- used an ECG to make the diagnosis
- assessed the presence/absence of risk factors such as CCF, hypertension, diabetes and history of prior cerebral ischaemia
- arranged appropriate further tests, e.g. FBC, U&Es, fasting glucose and lipids, TSH
- prescribed appropriately and explained the treatment using appropriate language
- referred for cardioversion

Test your theoretical knowledge

For each of the following statements, answer true (T) or false (F).

With respect to AF
1. AF is the most common arrhythmia in clinical practice
2. 2008 QOF points are awarded for having an AF register, confirming diagnosis by ECG or hospital specialist, and appropriate anticoagulation
3. The risk of stroke is increased by a factor of 10
4. A low dose beta blocker should be prescribed first-line to control rate
5. Patients should be anticoagulated before cardioversion

Relevant literature

NICE (June 2006). Atrial fibrillation: www.nice.org.uk/Guidance/CG36

Mock case 15 – A personal problem

Brief to the doctor

KB is a 17 year old boy who consults you because he has a 'personal problem'.

Patient summary

Name	KB
Date of birth (Age)	17 years
Social and family history	Single
Past medical history	Nil of note
Current medication	Nil
Investigations	None

Tasks for the doctor

In this case, the tasks are:
- to establish the reason for KB's attendance
- to identify and address KB's concerns and beliefs
- patient education

Brief to the patient – more about the patient

1. Profile:

- KB is a 17 year old college student
- he lives with his parents
- a friend has told him that a recent sexual partner, with whom KB had unprotected sex 4 weeks ago, has had genital herpes. This partner did not tell him about this. They only had sex on one occasion.
- he has not noticed any symptoms

2. He is seeing the doctor today because:

- he would like to know:
  - if you can catch herpes from someone who has no symptoms and not have any symptoms
  - if he should attend a GUM clinic
  - if he can just be given treatment without having any tests

3. Additional information:

- He is very embarrassed about attending the GP.
- He has been sexually active since age 15 years and has never had any STDs.
- His parents are unaware he is sexually active and he does not want them to know.
- He would prefer not to discuss his sex life and would like to concentrate on his specific questions.
- If the doctor suggests he should attend a GUM Clinic he will end the consultation, saying he will ask the GUM Clinic staff all the questions he would like answered. He will ask if he will have to be examined at the Clinic and what tests may be undertaken.
- If the doctor asks specifically:
  - he will tell him/her that he has had multiple partners since the age of 15 years
  - he uses condoms with partners he is unsure about, but if a partner says that they are 'clean' he will have unprotected sex because it 'feels much better'
- He is very concerned that he will be infected for ever and so will never be able to enjoy an unrestricted sex life again.
- If the doctor talks about being responsible or similar words, he will say 'you only live once' or 'being young is about having fun'.
- He will refuse to be examined.

Debrief

This case tests the doctor's ability to:

- take a sexual history
- deal with an embarrassed patient
- educate a patient about safe sex
- agree a safe management plan
- deal with a patient who refuses to be examined

Discuss how the doctor could, if needed, improve his performance. In particular, assess whether the doctor:

- dealt with the patient in an open, non-judgemental and relaxed manner
- recognised and dealt with the patient's embarrassment
- helped make the patient feel comfortable and at ease
- encouraged the patient to express his concerns
- answered the patient's questions using appropriate language
- encouraged the patient to consider the risks he was taking
- identified and dealt with the patient's refusal to be examined

Test your theoretical knowledge

For each of the following statements, answer true (T) or false (F).

1. The initial episode of genital herpes is lesions that rupture easily, heal within a week and may be associated with symptoms such as myalgia and fever
2. Suppressive antiviral therapy for 12 months does not reduce the number of recurrences in patients with frequent recurrences
3. There is evidence that genital herpes simplex virus (HSV) increases the risk of HIV infection
4. Most people with HSV infection have mild unrecognised or subclinical disease and may be unaware of their infection
5. Serological testing does not help make a diagnosis of HSV-2 infection

Relevant literature

Seri P, Barton SE. (2007) Genital herpes and its management. *BMJ*, **334:** 1048–1052.

Answers to "Test your theoretical knowledge" questions

Answers to Case 1

1. False – for vasomotor symptoms, consider a 2 week trial of paroxetine (20 mg daily)
2. True
3. False – Venlafaxine 37.5 mg twice a day is unlicensed for the treatment of menopausal flushing
4. True
5. False – ginseng, black cohosh, and red clover have oestrogenic properties and should not be used in women with contraindications to oestrogen (e.g. breast cancer)

Answers to Case 2

1. True
2. False – NICE guidelines require all of a list of criteria to be fulfilled before bariatric surgery can be recommended
3. True
4. False – NICE does not recommend use of bioimpedance, however, the National Obesity Forum guidelines do
5. True
6. True

Answers to Case 3

1. True
2. True
3. False – leave-on emollients should be prescribed in large quantities (250–500 g weekly)
4. True
5. False – NICE recommends that healthcare professionals review repeat prescriptions of products for children with atopic eczema at least once a year
6. False – topical tacrolimus is recommended, within its licensed indications, as an option for the second-line treatment of moderate to severe atopic eczema, in adults and children aged 2 years and older, that has not been controlled by topical corticosteroids
7. True
8. False – healthcare professionals should offer a 7–14 day trial of an age-appropriate sedating antihistamine to children aged 6 months or over during an acute flare of atopic eczema if sleep disturbance has a significant impact on the child or parents or carers

Answers to Case 4

1. False – it involves the common extensor muscle origin
2. True
3. True
4. False – trials have shown that corticosteroid injections relieve symptoms fairly quickly, but that this is not long-lasting
5. False – a multicentre European trial showed no benefit over placebo
6. True – some trials have shown benefit in tennis elbow and related conditions
7. True – both increase the torque and vibration the arm receives

Answers to Case 5

1. False – rest sprained ankles for 48 hours, after which active movement is encouraged
2. True
3. False – advise patients to improve balance by practising balancing on the injured leg with the eyes shut, once the pain has settled
4. True
5. False – more than 75% of ankle injuries are sprained ankles

Answers to Case 6

1. True
2. True
3. False – sensitivity is around 90%, but specificity is around 25%
4. True – but CT has a higher radiation dose
5. True – see 2007 Cochrane Review

Answers to Case 7

1. False – advise patients with gout to avoid purine-rich foods, such as liver, kidneys and seafood; bananas, chocolate and tuna are not a problem, see: http://arthritis.about.com/od/gout/a/foodstoeat.htm
2. False – consider prophylactic medication with allopurinol if a person is having two or more attacks of gout in a year
3. True
4. True
5. False – do not stop allopurinol during an acute attack of gout

Answers to Case 8

1. True – quinolones
2. True
3. False – both these features may be absent
4. True
5. False – there is hypervascularity with neovessel formation, collagen fibre disarray, but inflammatory cells are absent
6. False – evidence supports the use of heel-drop exercises, GTN patches, sclerosing injections and microcurrent therapy. While peritendinous corticosteroid injections have short-term pain-relieving benefits, they have no long-term effects.

Answers to Case 9

1. False – the pain is usually caused by collagen degeneration at the origin of the plantar fascia at the medial tubercle of the calcaneus
2. True
3. False – patients often notice pain at the beginning of activity that lessens or resolves as they warm up
4. False – patients with pes planus (low arches or flat feet) or pes cavus (high arches) are at increased risk for developing plantar fasciitis
5. True
6. True
7. False – with age, running shoes lose a significant portion of their shock absorption; getting a new pair of shoes may be helpful in decreasing pain
8. True

Answers to Case 10

1. True – anabolic steroids improve nitrogen utilization and promote positive nitrogen balance by the reversal of the catabolic process; intense training also tends to maintain a state of chronic catabolism
2. False – oral anabolic-androgenic steroids are usually undetectable 3–4 days after cessation, and their metabolites can be cleared from the body in 14 days; stanozolol has been detected in the urine of an athlete 4 months after use, while metabolites of nandrolone (an injectable anabolic-androgenic steroid) have been found in the urine up to 2 years after last reported use
3. True
4. True – insulin resistance and diminished glucose tolerance have been reported in powerlifters
5. True – anabolic-androgenic steroids have traditionally been used in 6–12 week cycles, often using more than one steroid at a time ("stacking"); users often "pyramid" use, moving from low starting doses to higher doses, and then "tapering" the dose down at the end of the cycle
6. True – they appear to increase arousal, self-confidence and pain threshold

Answers to Case 11

1. True
2. False – the WHO classifies anaemia in pregnant women, as an Hb < 11g/dl
3. False – if iron deficiency anaemia co-exists with a B12 or folate deficiency, the red cell distribution width (RDW) is increased
4. True
5. True
6. False – a 125 g can of sardines in tomato sauce contains more iron than two slices of lean roast beef
7. False – a 30 g bowl of branflakes contains three times more iron than a 30 g bowl of cornflakes

Answers to Case 12

1. True
2. False – about 90% of the risk for bowel cancer is thought to be due to dietary factors
3. False – trials have shown that the risk can be reduced by almost 50%
4. True – HNPCC is inherited as an autosomal dominant; familial polyposis coli accounts for 1% of cases
5. False – a single FOB is negative with up to 50% of cancers; the figure is about 30% if done on 3 consecutive days
6. True – refer to the July 2000 two week referral guidelines

Answers to Case 13

1. False – diarrhoea, cramping, abdominal pain, and fever within 2–5 days after exposure to the organism are symptoms of campylobacteriosis
2. False – some patients with campylobacteriosis may be asymptomatic
3. False – campylobacteriosis is often associated with the consumption of undercooked meat (especially poultry), unpasteurized milk, or untreated water
4. True
5. True
6. True
7. False – loperamide should be avoided in people with severe symptoms or dysentery because of the risk of precipitating ileus or toxic megacolon

Answers to Case 14

1. False – approximately 80% are asymptomatic
2. True
3. False – bacterial orchitis rarely occurs without an associated epididymitis and unilateral testicular oedema occurs in 90% of cases
4. True
5. True

Answers to Case 15

1. False – enuresis is the involuntary discharge of urine by day or night or both, in a child aged 5 years or older, in the absence of congenital or acquired defects of the nervous system or urinary tract
2. False – as many as 70% of children with nocturnal enuresis have a positive family history of childhood bedwetting
3. True
4. True
5. True
6. True
7. False – the only investigations required in primary nocturnal enuresis are urinalysis and urine culture to exclude diabetes mellitus and a urinary tract infection

8. False – do not restrict fluids; the child should have about eight drinks a day, spaced out throughout the day, the last one about 1 hour before bed
9. False – enuresis alarms, the first-line treatment in motivated children over 7 years, come in vibrating or sound modes; the vibrating alarm is preferable in children who share rooms or who are deaf
10. True

Answers to Case 16

1. True
2. True
3. False – it doubles the relative risk
4. True
5. False – NICE guidelines: localised intermediate risk prostate cancer can be treated with radical surgery, radical radiotherapy or active surveillance. Men with high risk localised cancer should be offered radical prostatectomy or external beam radiotherapy. Hormonal treatment is not routinely recommended for men with biochemical relapse after radical treatment unless they also have symptomatic local disease progression, or proven metastases, or a PSA level that has doubled in less than 3 months.

Answers to Case 17

1. False – dyspnoea, chest pain, or haemoptysis are symptoms of pulmonary embolism
2. False – a positive Homan's sign is pain in the calf or popliteal region on passive abrupt, forceful dorsiflexion of the ankle with the knee in a flexed position.
3. True
4. True
5. False – D-dimer assays are more sensitive for proximal than distal DVT, probably because proximal thromboses have a greater volume than distal thromboses
6. False – D-dimer levels can fall significantly after heparin is given
7. False – repeat ultrasonography is indicated in people with a negative initial ultrasound if they are at moderate to high risk for DVT and the D-dimer test was positive
8. False – one of the differential diagnoses of a DVT is a ruptured Baker's cyst, which is a cyst that forms in the popliteal fossa from an outpouching of synovial membrane of the knee joint

Answers to Case 18

1. False – 81% are venous
2. True
3. False – skin pigmentation and varicose veins suggest a venous cause, while cold, shiny hairless skin suggests an arterial cause
4. True
5. False – ulcers should be cleaned by gentle irrigation to prevent damaging the wound bed

6. False – graduated compression bandages should not be used if the ABPI suggests significant arterial disease
7. True – these patients may require surgery or angiography
8. False – antibiotics have little effect on wound healing and should not be used to treat organisms that have colonised a wound that are not causing clinical signs or symptoms of infection

Answers to Case 19

1. True
2. False – hoarseness due to hypothyroidism is unlikely to resolve with thyroxine treatment
3. True
4. False – if hoarseness persists for more than 6 weeks, refer to an ENT surgeon to inspect the vocal cords to exclude oropharyngeal malignancy
5. False – the effect of inhaled steroids on hoarseness is dose-related

Answers to Case 20

1. False – a 2-week washout period is required
2. True
3. True
4. True
5. False – UK prevalence is just under 30%

Answers to Mock case 1

1. True
2. True
3. False – hot flushes are often blamed for patients' sleep problems; however, results of polysomnographic studies have been inconclusive
4. False – postmenopausal women experience a decline in melatonin and growth hormone levels, both of which affect sleep
5. True
6. False – an FSH level >40 IU/l is often used as a marker of menopausal changes
7. True

Answers to Mock case 2

1. True – the most important allergens are indoor allergens such as house dust mite and pet allergens and outdoor allergens such as pollens
2. False – in population studies, about 40% of cases of chronic rhinoconjunctivitis are not sensitised to any allergen
3. False – there is no evidence for this (see de Groot *et al.* (2007) *BMJ*, **335**: 985–988)
4. True – occurs in 17–23% of patients, although it is also common (10–15%) in patients treated with placebo in clinical trials and so may be caused by local trauma from the nozzle of the spray rather than the drug itself
5. True – also beta blockers, NSAIDs and local decongestants

Answers to Mock case 3

1. True
2. False – many women with this condition are obese and have a higher prevalence of sleep apnoea than is observed in the general population
3. False – oligo- or anovulation or clinical and/or biochemical signs of hyperandrogenism are two of the three criteria diagnostic of PCOS; a raised luteinising hormone/follicle-stimulating hormone ratio is no longer a diagnostic criteria for PCOS owing to its inconsistency
4. True
5. True
6. False – orlistat and sibutramine have been shown to significantly reduce body weight and hyperandrogenism in women with PCOS
7. True

Answers to Mock case 4

1. False – over 80% of cancer pains can be effectively managed using analgesic drugs
2. False – the National Council for Palliative Care reports that nausea and vomiting occurs in 15–30% of patients commencing opioids
3. True – see National Council for Palliative Care guidelines
4. True
5. False – but guidelines advise also prescribing gastro-protective agents to all patients

Answers to Mock case 5

1. True
2. False – in resistant ovary syndrome, the ovaries contain many primordial follicles which are resistant to the action of gonadotrophins
3. False – prolactinomas will commonly shrink with medical therapy, but large tumours that affect vision may need surgical treatment. Other tumours of the pituitary, hypothalamus, ovary, and adrenal glands usually require surgery
4. True
5. False – estradiol levels are of limited usefulness, as they vary considerably even in a woman with amenorrhoea
6. True
7. True

Answers to Mock case 6

1. True
2. False – routine radiography is not recommended
3. False – although PEG is less likely to produce side effects such as abdominal pain and flatulence than lactulose
4. True – intermittent use is therefore recommended
5. True

Answers to Mock case 7

1. False – asking a person how much alcohol they drink has a low sensitivity for diagnosing an alcohol problem
2. False – the association between signs (tremor of the hands and tongue, and excessive capillarisation of the skin and conjunctivae) and increased alcohol intake has not been thoroughly investigated
3. True
4. False – the CAGE questionnaire is less sensitive than the AUDIT questionnaire in detecting hazardous drinking
5. True
6. False – fatty liver is present in 90% of persistently heavy drinkers
7. True

Answers to Mock case 8

1. True
2. True
3. False – if the pregnancy is very early, the ectopic might not be clear on a transvaginal scan, so a repeat scan is done a few days later
4. False – most ectopic pregnancies can be treated with planned but urgent surgery rather than requiring sudden emergency treatment
5. False – if an ectopic pregnancy is diagnosed early and there are few symptoms, it can sometimes be treated with methotrexate (unlicensed use) instead of surgery

Answers to Mock case 9

1. True
2. False – routine use of home monitoring devices in primary care is not currently recommended because their value has not been adequately established
3. False – offer drug therapy to patients at raised cardiovascular risk (10-year risk of CVD of 20% or more, or existing CVD or target organ damage) with persistent blood pressure of more than 140/90 mmHg
4. False – in black Afro-Caribbean (but not Asian) patients, the first choice for initial therapy should be either a calcium-channel blocker or a thiazide-type diuretic
5. True
6. True

Answers to Mock case 10

1. True
2. False – coeliac disease characteristically causes inflammatory changes in the duodenum and jejunum, however, any organ system can be affected
3. True
4. False – serological testing should be the first investigation with duodenal biopsy for those who are seropositive

5. False – false-negative serology occurs in 5–10% of cases with anti-endomysial antibodies (EmA) and for anti-transglutaminase antibodies (TGA) using human recombinant antigen
6. True
7. True

Answers to Mock case 11

1. False – allergy to cows' milk is the most common food allergy in childhood, affecting 2–7% of babies under 1 year old
2. True
3. True
4. False – children usually grow out of milk allergy by the age of three, but about one-fifth of children who have an allergy to cows' milk will still be allergic to it as adults
5. True
6. False – the allergic reaction can be to whole milk, or to casein or to whey
7. True
8. False – heat treatment doesn't affect casein, so someone who is allergic to casein will probably react to all types of milk and milk products

Answers to Mock case 12

1. False – seven consecutive doses of COC are required to inhibit ovulation; subsequent doses maintain anovulation
2. False – progestogen-only pills (POPs), containing norgestrel, desogestrel, levonorgestrel, norethisterone, or etynodiol diacetate, work by thickening cervical mucus, delaying ovum transport, inhibiting ovulation, and providing an endometrium hostile to implantation
3. False – the formulations of the progestogen-only injectables slowly release the active components and provide effective therapeutic levels for an extended period: 12 weeks for depot medroxyprogesterone acetate, and 8 weeks for nerethisterone enantate
4. True
5. True
6. False – most women (>75%) will continue to ovulate while using the levonorgestrel-releasing intrauterine system (IUS)
7. True

Answers to Mock case 13

1. False – treatment for the primary and secondary prevention of CVD should be initiated with simvastatin 40 mg
2. False – opportunistic assessment should not be the main strategy used in primary care to identify CVD risk in unselected people
3. False – the Framingham risk equation should not be used for people who are already considered at high risk of CVD because of familial hypercholesterolaemia, other monogenic disorders of lipid metabolism, or diabetes

4. False – the estimated CVD risk should be increased by a factor of 1.5 in people with a first-degree relative with a history of premature CHD (age at onset younger than 55 in fathers, sons or brothers or younger than 65 in mothers, daughters or sisters)
5. True
6. False – people at high risk of, or with, CVD should be advised to take 30 minutes of physical activity a day, of at least moderate intensity, at least 5 days a week
7. True
8. True
9. True
10. True

Answers to Mock case 14

1. True – reported as 5% of >75 year olds
2. True
3. False – stroke risk rises by 6, except in the presence of rheumatic heart disease when the risk increases by a factor of 18
4. True
5. True – reduces the risk of thromboembolism from around 6% to 1–2%

Answers to Mock case 15

1. False – lesions do rupture easily, leaving painful erosions and ulcers, and the initial episode may be accompanied by systemic symptoms, but healing of uncomplicated lesions takes 2–4 weeks
2. False – it reduces the number of recurrences by 70–80% in such patients
3. True
4. True
5. False – type-specific serology testing has sensitivity and specificity

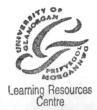

Learning Resources
Centre